Basic Trauma Life
Advanced Prehosp

D0537584

Publishing Director: David Culverwell
Acquisitions Editor: Richard Weimer
Production Editor / Text Design: Sandra Tamburrino
Art Director / Cover Design: Don Sellers, AMI
Assistant Art Director: Bernard Vervin
Manufacturing Director: John Komsa

Indexer: Leah Kramer
Typesetter: Port City Press, Inc., Baltimore, MD
Printer: R. R. Donnelley & Sons Co., Harrisonburg, VA
Typefaces: Caledonia (text), Bodoni (display)

Basic Trauma Life Support
Advanced Prehospital Care

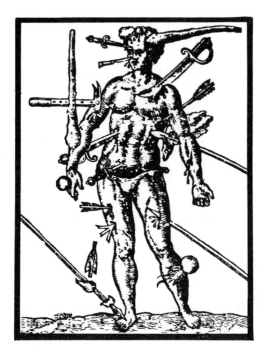

John E. Campbell, MD

Alabama Chapter, American College of
Emergency Physicians

Brady Communications Company, Inc., Bowie, MD 20715
A Prentice-Hall Publishing Company

Basic Trauma Life Support: Advanced Prehospital Care

Library of Congress Cataloging in Publication Data

Campbell, John E., 1943–
  Basic trauma life support.

  Bibliography: p.
  Includes index.
  1. Life support systems (Critical care). 2. Traumatology. 3. Medical emergencies. I. Title. [DNLM: 1. Emergency Medical Services. 2. Wounds and Injuries. 3. Allied Health Personnel. WX 215 C188b]
  RC86.7.C34   1985   617'.1026   84–14567

ISBN 0-89303-361-8

Prentice-Hall of Australia, Pty., Ltd., *Sydney*
Prentice-Hall Canada, Inc., Scarborough, *Ontario*
Prentice-Hall Hispanoamericana, S.A., *Mexico*
Prentice-Hall of India Private Limited, *New Delhi*
Prentice-Hall International, Inc., *London*
Prentice-Hall of Japan, Inc., *Tokyo*
Prentice-Hall of Southeast Asia Pte. Ltd., *Singapore*
Editora Prentice-Hall Do Brasil LTDA., *Rio de Janeiro*
Whitehall Books, Limited, Petone, *New Zealand*

Printed in the United States of America

88 89 90 91 92 93 94 95   6 7 8 9 10

This course was inspired by and is dedicated to my friend and mentor, Dr. Doyle C. Haynes. Not only is he nationally recognized as a trauma surgeon and teacher, but more importantly, when needed in the emergency department, he always appears faster than a speeding bullet. . .

Contents

Chapters

Skill Stations

Special thanks are in order to those whose help and encouragement contributed so much to the development of this manual. In particular, the staff of Southeast Alabama EMS, the Regional Education Department at East Alabama Medical Center, Alabama ACEP, and the Lee County EMT Association all worked as teammates in the endeavor. Dave Nathan and Barbara Dicey provided invaluable assistance in correcting the manual. I am especially grateful to my wife and children for tolerating me during this period.

This book is designed to be part of an organized 2-day, hands-on course. There are slides and an Instructor's Guide to be used with this book. This course is monitored and certified in each state, usually by the state chapter of American College of Emergency Physicians in conjunction with a regional state EMS agency. If you do not know who to contact in your state to arrange a certified course, you may obtain this information from:

National Office, BTLS
3840 Interstate Court, Suite A
Montgomery, Alabama 36109
Phone 205-277-0911

Introduction

The day I took the American College of Surgeon's excellent *Advanced Trauma Life Support* course, I realized that the concept of a hands-on course about trauma was too important to teach to physicians only. The traumatized patient must reach the emergency department alive for the physician to bring his advanced skills into action.

This *Basic Trauma Life Support* course was introduced in August of 1982. After 18 months and approximately 20 courses, this revised manual was completed. We have attempted to make changes that are more practical to the real environment of the prehospital situation. The *Advanced Trauma Life Support* course (for physicians) was used as a model so that the surgeon, emergency physician, trauma nurse, and EMT will be thinking and acting along the same lines. There are differences, of course, because the prehospital situation is very different from the hospital situation. Different priorities must apply. The term *"basic trauma life support"* is not to suggest that advanced life support procedures are not used in the field, but rather to distinguish the support in the field from the advanced surgical procedures used in the hospital care of the trauma victim.

This course is designed for the advanced EMT, paramedic, and trauma nurse who must initially evaluate and stabilize the trauma patient. Since this is a critical time in the management of these patients, this course is intended to teach the skills necessary for rapid assessment, resuscitation, stabilization, and transport. It also stresses those conditions which cannot be stabilized in the field and thus require immediate transport. It is recognized that there is more than one acceptable way to manage most situations, and the one described here is not the only way. You should have your Medical Control physician go over the material and give you his advice as to how you do things in your area.

The primary objectives of the course are to teach you the correct sequence of evaluation and the techniques of resuscitation and stabilization and to give you enough practical training so that you can perform these drills rapidly and efficiently, thus giving your patient the greatest chance of arriving at the emergency department in time for definitive care to be lifesaving.

Chapter 1

Initial Evaluation of the Trauma Victim

It is heartbreaking to see a life lost, especially if it happens because treatment is instituted too little and too late. In the severely injured patient, time is of the essence. Evaluation and resuscitation actually begin simultaneously. Thus, a habit of assessing and treating every trauma patient in a preplanned logical and sequential manner must be developed.

Remember, as the first person treating the patient, you have a profound effect on his eventual outcome: he may live or die as the result of the speed and capability of your actions.

Philosophy of Rapid Trauma Management: "The Golden Hour"

Dr. R. Adams Cowley, through his pioneer work in trauma management at the Maryland Institute of Emergency Medicine, found that multiple trauma victims who received definitive care *within 60 minutes* of their injuries had the best chance for recovery. The overall mortality rate (15% to 20%) for multiple trauma victims doubled for every hour lost in receiving that care. Again, this stresses the urgency of getting a victim to the operating room within the hour following his injury to maximize his chance for recovery: a task which requires teamwork and optimal performance in all phases of prehospital management. The "golden hour," once lost, cannot be bought back at any price.

Rapid management does not mean simply racing down the highway at breakneck speed, throwing the victim into the back of the ambulance, and racing to the nearest emergency room. The trauma victim has the best chance for survival if you properly perform your duties during the six stages of an ambulance call. These are outlined below.

I. **Predispatch**
   This is the first (and often ignored) stage of prehospital care. Lifesaving care cannot be given if you cannot find the accident, if you do not know the shortest route, or if your ambulance or rescue

1

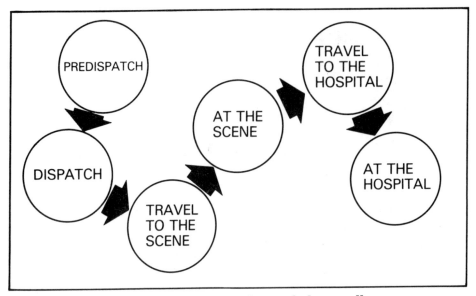

Figure 1-1. Six stages of an ambulance call.

vehicle is not ready to respond. Before you begin taking ambulance calls, you must learn the area that you serve. You should know the streets and highways well enough to immediately pick out the shortest route and should keep in mind an alternate route in case traffic conditions, weather, or other conditions make it unwise to take the shortest route. Fast driving will not make up for lack of map training. Between runs the vehicle must be checked, fueled, and restocked immediately.

II. **Dispatch**
The ambulance crew must have the proper information to rapidly respond to a call:
   A. The exact nature of the call: What happened? How many victims? Are there dangers at the scene? Will special equipment be needed?
   B. The exact location of the call: This cannot be overemphasized. If an exact address cannot be given, get directions that are as precise as possible.
   C. A call back number: This can be invaluable if you have trouble locating the scene of the accident. Units equipped with Radio Telephone Switch Station (RTSS) can call back for more information about the accident while they are responding.

III. **Travel to the Scene**
Make a rapid yet careful response using your best judgment concerning the fastest route. Obtain the necessary information from the dispatcher (or from a call back to the scene) so you can make decisions about backup help and equipment needed.

IV. **Actions at the Scene**

You must make a quick assessment of the overall situation. Park the ambulance as close as possible, keeping in mind the dangers (i.e., traffic, fire, explosion, powerlines) of the scene. Quickly note the apparent mechanisms of injury. Be aware of the number of victims and call for help if needed. As a general rule, one ambulance is needed for every seriously injured victim. Begin evaluation of the most seriously injured victim first. Stabilize and package the victims using the priority plan. Be rapid but careful and *gentle*. Rough handling aggravates injuries.

V. **Travel to the Hospital**

Select the most suitable route and hospital according to your local protocols. The most experienced EMT should remain at the victim's side and provide continuous monitoring. Notify Medical Control if the victim's condition deteriorates during transport. Notify the receiving facility of your estimated time of arrival and any special needs.

VI. **Actions at the Hospital**

You must continue your care until you are relieved by the emergency department staff; never leave a victim unattended. Report pertinent information about the victim to the nurse or physician in charge. This should include mechanisms of injury, observed and suspected injuries, procedures performed, and changes in condition. Remain as long as you are needed, but when no longer required, you should complete your run report and immediately prepare your vehicle for return to service.

Trauma Assessment

As you begin your evaluation, you must immediately categorize the victim into one of four groups:

C 1. *CPR:* This is for a victim in respiratory or cardiac arrest.

U̲ 2. *Unstable:* This patient will be in obvious shock and/or respiratory difficulty.

P̲ 3. *Potentially unstable:* This patient has borderline abnormal vital signs and is the most likely victim to be lost due to delayed and inadequate treatment.

S̲ 4. *Stable:* This patient has normal vital signs and no respiratory problems.

This CUPS categorization becomes most important when you have more than one victim and must decide who is to be transported first. Remember, the condition category may change from minute to minute, so you must continually reassess.

Assessment Priorities

Assessment and treatment priorities should be approached in this order:

1. Airway maintenance and control of cervical spine
2. Assessment of breathing and circulation
3. Control of hemorrhage
4. Treatment of shock
5. Evaluation for further injuries, including brief neurological examination and splinting of fractures
6. Transportation with continuous monitoring

These steps must be memorized until you can perform them in the correct sequence without stopping to think about what comes next. They are the ABCs of basic trauma life support. In brief, you are learning to do a rapid primary survey and resuscitation of vital functions, followed by a secondary survey. In some cases the primary survey may dictate rapid transport so that the secondary survey has to be done during transport or, in other cases, not until the patient arrives at the emergency department.

Patient Assessment Using the Priority Plan

Assessment begins immediately: often while the victim is being extricated. Always approach the victim from the head. Immediately and gently, but firmly, stabilize the neck in a neutral position. You must not release your hold on the neck until someone relieves you or a suitable stabilization device is applied. Once the neck is stabilized, the following procedures should be performed.

I. **Assess the Airway**
   A. Look, listen, and feel for movement of air.
   B. Open the mouth and clear the airway if necessary. If the airway is obstructed, use suction or instruments such as a laryngoscope and forceps. If the victim is on a backboard or a firm surface, you may use abdominal thrusts. Do not do back slaps on someone with a possible spinal injury. Because of this danger of spinal injury, the airway is handled differently in the trauma victim. You should *never* extend the neck to open the airway or turn the victim to do back slaps.

II. **Assess Breathing and Circulation**
   It is impractical to separate evaluation of breathing and heartbeat since you must check both as you quickly look, listen, and feel the neck and chest. There is a great deal of information to be gained

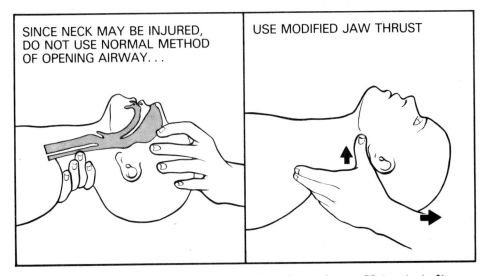

SINCE NECK MAY BE INJURED, DO NOT USE NORMAL METHOD OF OPENING AIRWAY...

USE MODIFIED JAW THRUST

Figure 1-2. Opening airway using modified jaw thrust. Maintain in-line traction while pushing up on the angles of the jaw with your thumbs.

quickly when this examination is performed correctly. Remember, if the victim is not breathing, you should immediately give four quick breaths and then check for a carotid pulse. If there is no pulse, you must begin cardiopulmonary resuscitation. (The trauma arrest will be discussed later.)

After you have stabilized the neck and opened the airway with a jaw thrust, you should proceed with evaluation of breathing and circulation in the following manner.

A. Place your face over the victim's mouth so you can judge both the rate and quality of respiration. Is respiration too fast or too slow? Is the victim moving an adequate volume of air when he breathes? Remember, several chest injuries (tension pneumothorax, sucking chest wounds, flail chest) present with inability to move air in spite of an open airway. If there is *any* difficulty with respiration, have one of your team members administer oxygen.

B. As you hold the neck stable and open the airway by pushing upward on the angles of the jaw with your thumbs, you will find that it is simple to feel the carotid pulse with your index finger.

C. As soon as you have noted the rate and quality of respiration, look quickly at the neck and notice if the trachea is in the midline, if the neck veins are flat or distended, or if there is discoloration or swelling. A Philadelphia cervical collar (or other suitable extrication collar or stabilization device) may be applied by another member of the team at this time. You

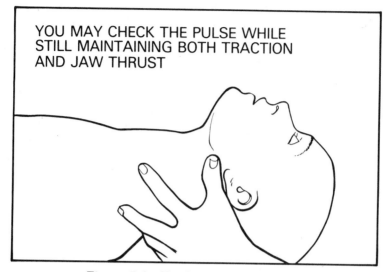

YOU MAY CHECK THE PULSE WHILE STILL MAINTAINING BOTH TRACTION AND JAW THRUST

Figure 1-3. Checking carotid pulse.

are now free to release the neck and continue with the examination. (Cervical stabilization will be covered in greater detail later.)

D. Now look, listen, and feel the chest. If there is any difficulty with respiration, the chest must be bared for examination: this is no time for modesty; chest injuries often kill quickly. Look for sucking chest wounds, flail segment, bruising, or deformity. Note if the ribs rise with respiration or if there is only diaphragmatic breathing. Listen for breath sounds and heart sounds. Feel for instability of ribs or subcutaneous emphysema. If breath sounds are decreased or absent on one side, you should percuss the chest to see if it is hyperresonant (pneumothorax) or dull (hemothorax). By this time one of your team members should have determined the blood pressure.

III. **Stop any Bleeding**
One of your teammates should have done this already by the time you finish your evaluation of airway, breathing, and circulation. Almost all bleeding can be controlled by direct pressure; use gauze pads and bandages or ACE™ wraps. You may use air splints or military anti-shock trousers (MAST) to tamponade bleeding; tourniquets may be needed in *rare* situations. If a dressing becomes blood soaked, add more dressings and wrap tighter; do not remove the blood soaked dressings. Do not use clamps to stop bleeders—you may cause injury to other structures (nerves run with arteries).

IV. **Assess for Shock**
To determine if shock exists, look at the whole patient, not only his blood pressure. Is the victim pale, diaphoretic, confused, combative, weak, or thirsty? All of these signs of hemorrhagic shock

may appear before a drop in blood pressure occurs. Remember that[the victim with spinal shock will not have tachycardia, vasoconstriction, or diaphoresis.]Note the etiology of the shock if possible[If shock is present, treat with oxygen, MAST, and intravenous fluids.]

V. **Secondary Survey**

At this point you have taken care of the resuscitation of vital functions. Now you should be completing your examination and preparing the victim for transport. Make a habit of beginning again at the head and working quickly to the feet, checking not only for bone and soft tissue injury, but also rechecking the vital signs. Wounds should be covered and fractures splinted. A brief neurological examination and abdominal examination should be done at this time. The victim should be log-rolled (stabilize the neck while doing this) and a backboard slid underneath. This is a good time to quickly check the back for injury. If the victim required treatment for shock, it is usually more practical to place the victim on the spine board as you apply the anti-shock trousers. If you do apply anti-shock trousers, you must first check the abdomen, pelvis, and lower extremities since you cannot see them after the trousers are in place. Often, you will find that you have done most of the secondary survey by the time you have initiated treatment for shock. It is still a good idea to do a quick head-to-toes examination and recheck everything. This takes only a few seconds and often picks up something overlooked.

Important Points in the Secondary Survey

A. Brief neurological examination
  1. Level of consciousness:
    A̲ Alert
    V̲ Responds to verbal stimuli
    P̲ Responds to pain
    U̲ Unresponsive
  2. Motor: Can he move fingers and toes?
  3. Sensation: Can he feel you when you touch him? Does he respond to pain?
  4. Pupils: Are they equal or unequal? Do they respond to light?
B. Abdominal examination: Look for signs of blunt or penetrating trauma. Feel for tenderness. Listening for bowel sounds is usually a waste of time. If the abdomen is distended and painful or even just painful on palpation, you can expect the victim to be bleeding internally. Be prepared for hemorrhagic shock!
C. Assess and splint fractures: Be sure to check distal sensation

and pulses on all fractures. Record these. Do this examination before and after straightening any fracture. Angulated fractures of the upper extremities are usually best splinted as found. Most fractures of the lower extremities are straightened by using a traction splint. (Splinting will be covered in another chapter and also in a skill station.)

D. Maxillofacial trauma
  1. Injuries to the face that do not obstruct the airway may be treated after the patient's life-threatening injuries are treated (up to 10 days later).
  2. The important thing to remember is that all patients with maxillofacial trauma should be treated as if they have cervical spine injury until proven otherwise by x-ray.
  3. All of these patients must have immobilization of the cervical spine.

E. Obtain a history of the injury
  1. Personal observation
  2. Bystanders
  3. Patient himself: Look for a Medic Alert tag in unconscious victims.

VI. **Transport**

A. Contact Medical Control
  1. Many times the need to secure the airway or start treatment of shock may necessitate your contacting Medical Control before all of the above steps are done. The more unstable the victim, the sooner you should contact Medical Control and the sooner transport should occur. If you work in a state with standing orders, you may not need to contact Medical Control until the victim is ready for transport.
  2. Procedure:
    a. Identify yourself; give your level of training and organization.
    b. Give the patient's approximate age, sex, nature of the injuries, vital signs, state of consciousness, and condition category (CUPS).
    c. Perform advanced life support as directed.
    d. Transport the patient to the facility named by Medical Control.
    e. Notify the facility of the estimated time of arrival (ETA), the condition of the patient, and any special needs on arrival.

B. If you are unable to perform a necessary resuscitative procedure or if the patient's condition is deteriorating in spite of your best efforts, you should load and go. Minutes are important—if you are not helping, you should be moving.

    C. Continuously monitor and reevaluate the patient.

    D. Contact Medical Control if the patient's condition deteriorates during transport.

    E. Accurately record what you see and what you do. Record changes in the patient's condition during transport; record the time MAST or tourniquet is applied. Extenuating circumstances or significant details should be noted in the comments or remarks section of the run report.

Summary

This is the content of the course in one chapter: a rapid, orderly, thorough examination of the trauma victim with priorities of examination and treatment always in mind. The continuous practice of approaching the patient in this way will allow you to concentrate on the patient rather than on trying to figure out what to do next. Optimum speed is achieved by teamwork. Teamwork is achieved only by practice. During the predispatch stage, you should plan regular exercises in patient evaluation in order to perfect each team member's role in the priority plan.

Chapter 2

Airway Maintenance and Ventilation

I. **Upper Airway**
The airway is the first priority in the evaluation of any sick or injured patient; if the patient is unable to exchange air, all other efforts at resuscitation are futile. The upper airway is separated from the lower airways by the vocal cords. In the field we can generally visualize and gain control of the upper airway, whereas injuries or obstruction of the lower airways often cannot be treated until the patient arrives at the hospital.

II. **Anatomy of Airway**
The tongue, pharynx, epiglottis, vallecula, vocal cords, and glottic opening are the key anatomical points of the upper airway with which you should become familiar. The lower airways are made up of the larynx, trachea, carina, bronchi, and lungs.

III. **Obstruction to Upper Airway**
   A. Tongue: This is the most common obstruction to the airway in an unconscious patient. The tongue attaches to the anterior mandible. One does not "stick" one's tongue out, but rather it is pulled out of the mouth by contraction of the genioglossus muscle. In the unconscious patient the tone is lost in the muscles of the tongue, and when the patient is in a supine position, the tongue is allowed to fall back and obstruct the upper airway. Since the tongue is attached to the mandible, lifting the mandible has the same effect as contracting the muscles: it pulls the tongue up and out of the pharynx.
   B. Foreign bodies: These include vomitus, blood, food, and dentures, among others. As you evaluate for an open airway, always clear the mouth and pharynx of these foreign bodies using your fingers or suction. You may not be able to remove blood or thick vomitus with suction; in this case, the victim must be log-rolled (stabilize the neck while doing this) into a face-down position to prevent aspiration and to allow gravity to help clear the upper airway.
   C. Edema: This includes edema of the glottic area or injury and spasm of the vocal cords. Direct injury to the soft tissue of

11

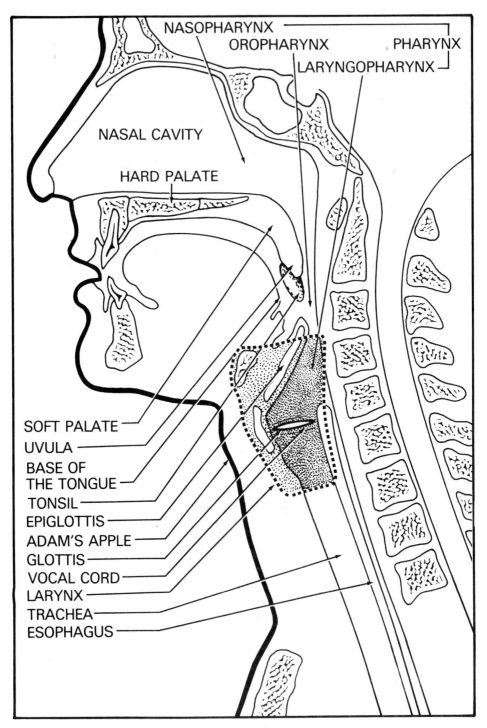

Figure 2-1. Upper airway.

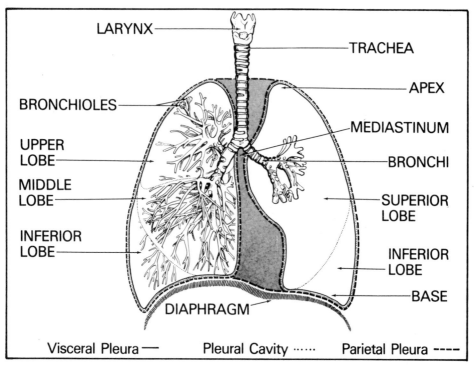

LARYNX

TRACHEA

APEX

BRONCHIOLES

MEDIASTINUM

UPPER LOBE

BRONCHI

MIDDLE LOBE

SUPERIOR LOBE

INFERIOR LOBE

INFERIOR LOBE

BASE

DIAPHRAGM

Visceral Pleura —   Pleural Cavity ······   Parietal Pleura ----

Figure 2-2. Lower airways.

the neck can cause rapid obstruction of the airway by swelling. This presents with stridor like that seen in epiglottitis, croup, and allergic edema of the vocal cords. Rapid endotracheal intubation (using a small tube: 6 or 6.5 mm I.D.) is the treatment of choice but may be impossible because of the following:

1. There is the likelihood of an intact gag reflex if the victim is conscious.
2. Edema is already too far advanced to see the landmarks or to pass a tube between the vocal cords.

An esophageal gastric tube airway (EGTA) is not helpful because it does not maintain an opening into the trachea. If the edema is advanced, this may be a situation in which nothing short of a cricothyroidotomy or even a tracheostomy will provide access to the lower airways, in which case you should immediately transport the patient.

IV. **Techniques for Opening Airway**
   A. Manual techniques to open the airway: Note that the standard advanced cardiac life support (ACLS) method of extending the neck to open the airway is *not* done in the trauma situation. If there is any chance of neck injury, one of the following techniques should be used.

1. Jaw thrust—modified: This is the method of choice for the trauma victim since it is the only one you can do while stabilizing the neck. The other methods require two rescuers to perform these tasks. When you place your hands on either side of the neck to hold traction, use your thumbs to push up on the angles of the mandible to open the airway. From this position you can also use your index fingers to check for a carotid pulse.

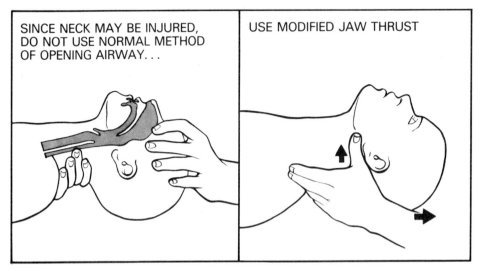

SINCE NECK MAY BE INJURED, DO NOT USE NORMAL METHOD OF OPENING AIRWAY. . .

USE MODIFIED JAW THRUST

Figure 2-3. Modified jaw thrust.

2. Chin lift: This requires two rescuers—one to stabilize the neck and the other to open the airway. The rescuer opening the airway uses his thumb to grasp the chin just below the lower lip while the fingers of that hand are placed underneath the anterior mandible and the chin is gently lifted. The chin lift can be used in connection with mouth-to-mouth breathing.
3. Jaw lift: This is the same as the chin lift except the thumb goes inside the mouth and grasps the lower incisors to lift the jaw. The disadvantages are as follows:
    a. You cannot do mouth-to-mouth breathing.
    b. Wet teeth are slippery.
    c. You may get bitten if the patient regains consciousness or has a seizure.
B. Mechanical methods to open the airway
    1. Oral airway: The oral airway is a semicircular apparatus of plastic or rubber. Its function is to hold the tongue forward and thus keep the airway open. Because of its shape, incorrect insertion can push the base of the tongue

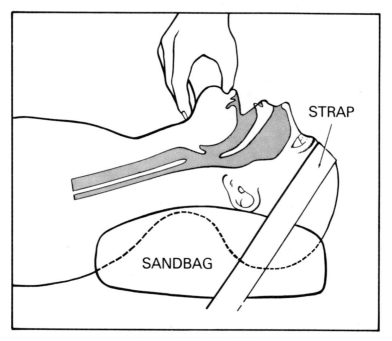

Figure 2-4. Chin lift.

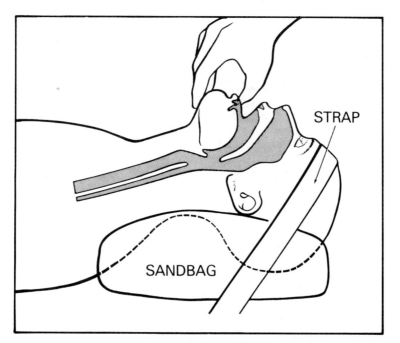

Figure 2-5. Jaw lift.

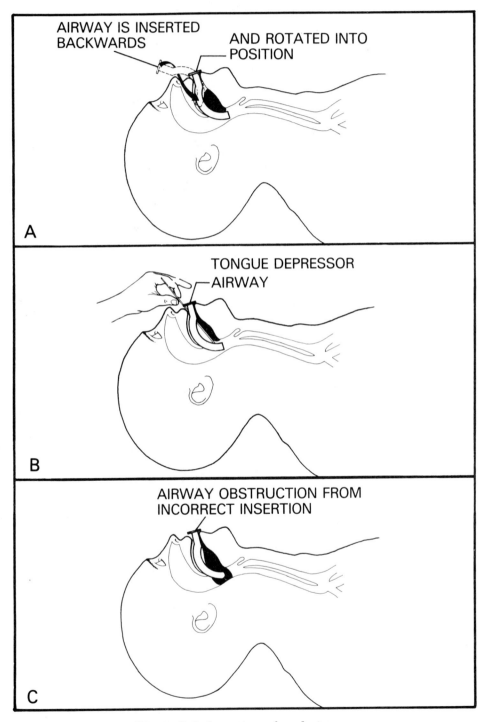

Figure 2-6. Insertion of oral airway.

down and obstruct the airway. There are two methods of insertion:

a. Insert the airway upside down until it reaches the posterior pharynx and then rotate it 180 degrees so that it slips behind the tongue.

b. Push the tongue out of the way with a tongue blade so that you can see that the device is inserted into the correct place.

Remember: The oral airway is reserved for use in the unconscious patient. Its use in a conscious patient will cause retching and vomiting.

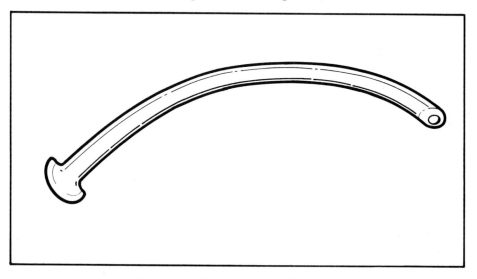

Figure 2-7. Nasopharyngeal airway.

2. Nasopharyngeal airway: This is a soft rubber or plastic tube about 6 inches in length. It is tolerated by the conscious patient, but suctioning cannot be accomplished well with this device. To insert it first lubricate it well, preferably with a lubricant that contains a local anesthetic. Insert it through one nostril into the posterior pharynx behind the tongue. The bevel goes toward the nasal septum. You will notice that the airway is made to go into the right nostril. In about 10% to 15% of the population, the septum is deviated so that you may not be able to insert it into the right nostril. To put it in the left nostril, turn the airway upside down so that the bevel is toward the septum, then insert the airway straight back through the nostril until you reach the posterior pharynx. At this point turn the airway over 180 degrees and insert it down the pharynx until it lies behind the tongue.

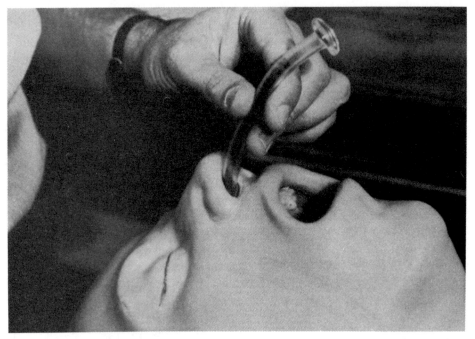

Figure 2-8. Insertion of nasopharyngeal airway into right nostril.

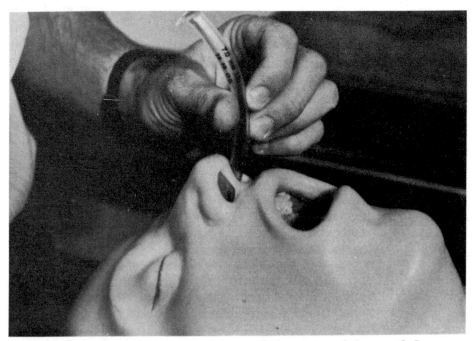

Figure 2-9a. Insertion of nasopharyngeal airway into left nostril. Insert upside down so bevel is toward the septum.

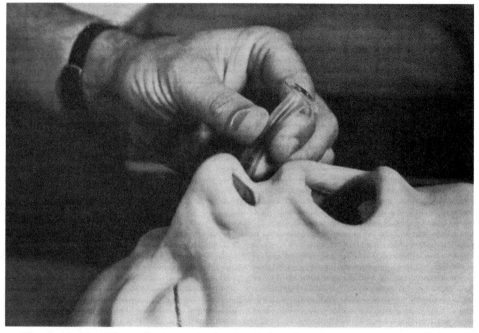

Figure 2-9b. When tip is to the back of the pharynx, rotate airway 180 degrees.

Remember: The opening through the nasal cavity goes straight back to the pharynx. It does not go upward. If you reach an obstruction, try the other side. If you try to force it, you may cause a nosebleed.

3. Esophageal obturator airway (EOA) and esophageal gastric tube airway (EGTA):
   a. The EOA is a plastic tube about 15 inches long. The distal end is sealed and there is a balloon near the tip that is blown up to seal the esophagus. The EOA performs two functions:
      1) It prevents stomach contents from getting up into the pharynx where they could be aspirated.
      2) It seals the esophagus so that air blown into the pharynx will enter the trachea and lungs.
   b. The EGTA performs the same functions as the EOA but has been improved by the addition of an opening in the tube through which a nasogastric tube can be inserted to aspirate the stomach contents. The EGTA and EOA are therefore ventilated through different openings in the mask. *Since the development of the EGTA, there is no reason to ever use an EOA. All EOAs should be replaced with the EGTA.* A further improvement of the EGTA can be made by replacing

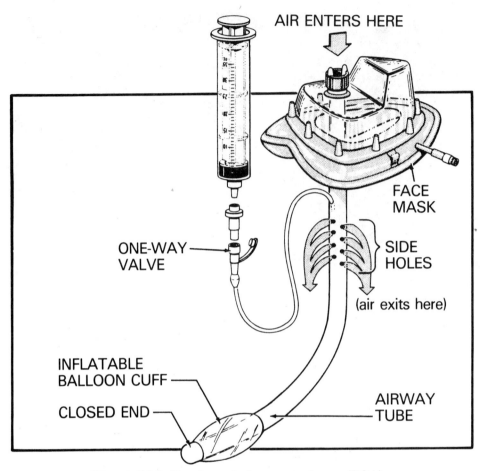

Figure 2-10. Esophageal obturator airway (EOA).

the EGTA tube with a #9 endotracheal tube; its 15-mm adapter will fit in the same hole as the EGTA tube adapter (it may require some trimming). The #9 endotracheal tube is approximately the same size and length as the EGTA tube and it will tolerate blowing up the balloon with 35 cc of air (at least a few times). The advantages of using the endotracheal tube with the EGTA are as follows:

1) The hole in the tube is larger so suctioning is easier.
2) It is cheaper to replace than replacing the whole EGTA.
3) If you inadvertently intubate the trachea while inserting the EGTA, you can remove the face

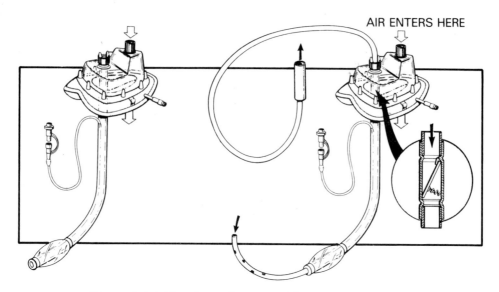

AIR ENTERS HERE

Figure 2-11. Esophageal gastric tube airway (EGTA).

mask and ventilate directly through the endotracheal tube.

c. EGTAs are for use only in unconscious patients. Because vomiting usually follows removal, an endotracheal tube must be inserted before removing the EGTA. If the patient with an EGTA regains consciousness first, you will have to remove the device, but you will not have to replace it with an endotracheal tube. However, you must be prepared for the patient to vomit when the tube is removed; log roll him on his side and have suction ready so that he does not aspirate.

d. EGTAs are for short-term use only: 2 hours or less. They are not for use in a patient with a history of corrosive ingestion or esophageal disease or in a patient under 14 to 15 years of age. You should also not use an EGTA if there is injury or bleeding in the upper airway because the balloon seals only the esophagus. Blood, teeth, or other foreign bodies can be aspirated into the trachea. The primary indication for use of the EGTA in the trauma victim is when you have difficulty with endotracheal intubation.

e. Technique for inserting the EGTA: Grasp the lower jaw with the thumb and forefinger, pull slightly, and insert the tube blindly through the mouth and pharynx. The tube will follow the curvature of the pharynx and usually pass into the esophagus. The neck should

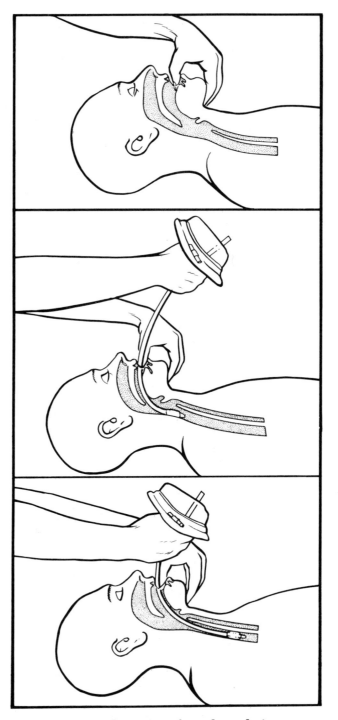

Figure 2-12. Insertion of esophageal airway.

not be extended. Advance the tube until the mask is seated on the face. When this is accomplished, the cuff will lie below the level of the carina. There is always the possibility that the tube may enter the trachea, so you must now blow into the airway (with mouth or bag-valve device) and both observe for chest expansion and listen for bilateral breath sounds. If air is entering the chest, you may then blow up the cuff with up to 35 mL of air. If air is not entering the chest, you must immediately remove the EGTA and ventilate the patient several times before another attempt is made to insert the airway. Once the EGTA is properly inserted, you must maintain an airtight seal with the face mask in order to ventilate. This is usually a two-man procedure. One man holds the face mask while the other ventilates the patient.

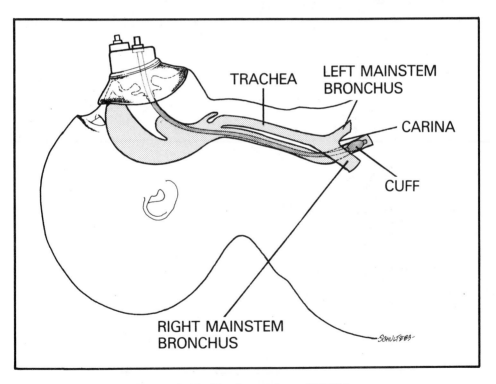

Figure 2-13. Final position of EGTA.

f. Review of "Rules for the EGTA":
  1) Use it only on an unconscious patient.
  2) Do not use it in children under 14 to 15 years of age.

3) Use it only until an endotracheal tube can be safely inserted (2 hours or less).

4) Do not remove it from the unconscious patient without first inserting an endotracheal tube.

5) If the patient regains consciousness, you must remove the tube (do *not* insert endotracheal tube) but take precautions to prevent aspiration of vomitus (log roll entire body to the side and suction as you remove).

6) Check the chest carefully to be sure air is entering both lungs before blowing up the cuff.

7) Be sure you get a good seal on the face mask.

8) Do not use it if there is continued bleeding of the upper airway.

4. Endotracheal intubation:

a. The endotracheal tube (ET tube) is a plastic tube, available in various sizes, that is inserted directly into the trachea. The adult sizes have a cuff at the distal end to seal the trachea from aspiration of foreign material—from either the stomach or the upper air-

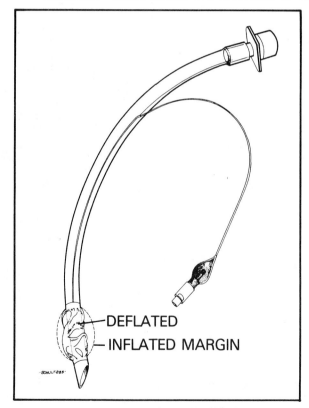

DEFLATED

INFLATED MARGIN

Figure 2-14. Endotracheal tube.

way. Each ET tube is equipped with a standard 15-mm adapter to fit bag-valve devices. This method of securing the airway is by far the best. In most trauma victims it may be done without difficulty once the neck is stabilized in a neutral position. With practice, most rescuers find they can intubate just as easily without the neck being extended. The main problem in using the ET tube in the trauma victim is that three people may be needed to correctly perform endotracheal intubation. One person must stabilize the neck from below, another is usually needed to press down on the cricoid cartilage, and a third is needed to insert the endotracheal tube.

b. Technique for inserting the ET tube (to be covered again in Skill Station 2):

1) If you are using a cuffed tube, attach a 5- or 10-cc syringe and blow up the cuff to be sure it does not leak.

2) Insert a wire guide and bend to the approximate configuration of the pharynx.

3) Have your suction ready.

4) Pick up the laryngoscope handle with your left hand and the appropriate blade with your right hand.

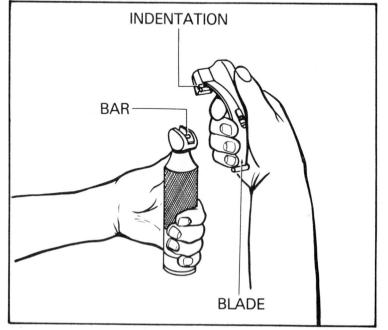

INDENTATION

BAR

BLADE

Figure 2-15. Attachment of laryngoscope blade to handle. Blade snaps into place when engaged properly.

5) Attach the blade to the handle by inserting the U-shaped indentation of the blade into the small bar at the end of the handle. Hold the blade parallel to the handle to do this.

6) When the indentation is aligned with the bar, press the blade forward and snap into place.

7) Lower the blade until it is at a right angle to the handle. The light should come on. If it does not, see if the bulb is tight and/or the batteries need replacement. (This should be done on a daily basis so you do not have to spend valuable time fixing it at the scene of the accident).

8) Maintain stabilization of the neck in a neutral position. This should be done from below.

9) Suction the pharynx if necessary.

10) Insert the blade into the mouth on the right side, moving the tongue to the left. Follow the natural contour of the pharynx, lifting the tongue (not prying) until you can see the glottic opening.

11) If you are using a straight blade, insert it until you can see the epiglottis; lift up with the tip of the blade so that you are looking at the vocal cords and glottic opening. You may have to have

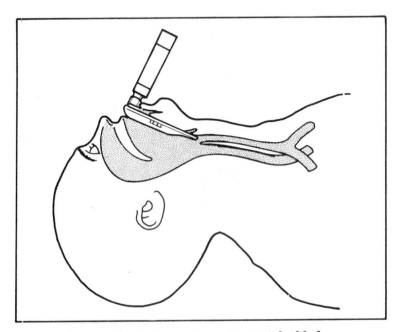

Figure 2-16a. Laryngoscope: straight blade.

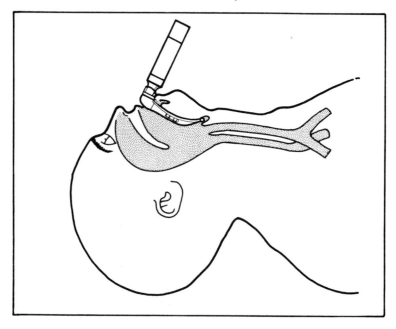

Figure 2-16b. Laryngoscope: curved blade.

someone press down gently on the cricoid cartilage so that you can see the cords well.

12) If you are using a curved blade, insert the tip into the vallecula and lift up. This will lift the epiglottis and expose the cords and glottic opening. You may have to have someone press down gently on the cricoid cartilage so that you can see the cords well.

13) Insert the ET tube with your right hand from the right corner of the mouth. As soon as you see the tip pass through the cords, insert the tube only far enough to pass the cuff, then stop and ventilate through the tube while listening to each side of the chest with a stethoscope to be sure air is entering both lungs. If you hear breath sounds on both sides, inflate the cuff with 5 cc to 10 cc of air and secure the tube. If you have inserted the tube too far, it will usually go into the right mainstem bronchus, so if you hear breath sounds only on the right, you should pull the tube back ½ inch at a time until you hear bilateral breath sounds. If you hear no breath sounds, you are in the esophagus and must remove the tube, ventilate the patient by another method for a few moments, and try again.

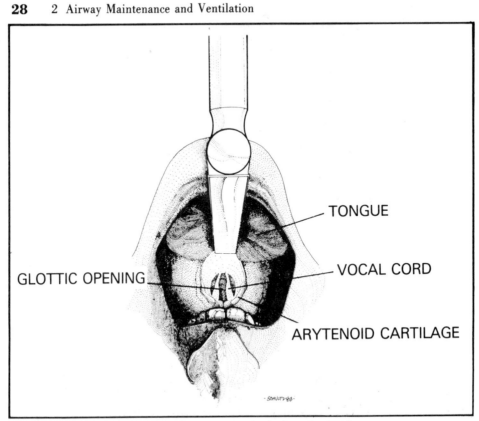

TONGUE

VOCAL CORD

GLOTTIC OPENING

ARYTENOID CARTILAGE

Figure 2-17a. Insertion of straight blade.

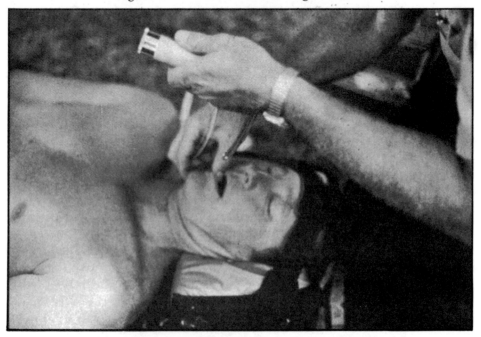

Figure 2-17b. Insertion of straight blade.

14) Secure the tube well with tape so that it does not inadvertently slip out of the trachea or slide too far down. You must frequently listen for breath sounds to be sure the ET tube stays in place.

15) Endotracheal intubation requires much practice to master. The greatest danger to the patient is wasting too much time attempting the difficult procedure. Time is precious: if you cannot intubate in two attempts, use another method but do not hold up the patient's transport. Do not interrupt ventilation for more than 15 to 20 seconds per attempt.

5. Surgical methods of treating upper airway obstruction: Tracheostomy, surgical cricothyroidotomy, and needle cricothyroidotomy are all moderately difficult surgical procedures that are fraught with a high rate of complications even when done in the controlled environment of the hospital. They are beyond the scope of a basic course.

V. **Breathing—Ventilation**
  A. Mouth-to-mouth
    1. This is still the superior method of ventilation because of the following:
      a. You can give a larger volume of air with each breath than with a bag-valve device.
      b. You can feel better the amount of resistance in the airway.
      c. You can get a better seal on the mouth than with a face mask.
      d. It can be done adequately by one rescuer.
    2. The disadvantages of mouth-to-mouth ventilation are as follows:
      a. The face is often covered with blood or vomitus. It takes extreme dedication to do mouth-to-mouth under these circumstances.
      b. It is difficult to give oxygen-enriched air mixtures. You can hold an oxygen line next to your mouth, but this does not provide a large increase over room air.
      c. This is a tiring procedure, and you may hyperventilate if you continue too long.
  B. Mouth-to-mask: The pocket mask is a very useful device that can be used to prevent direct contact of your mouth with the patient's nose and mouth. You can ventilate well as long as you maintain a good seal on the patient's face. This device has a nipple to which an oxygen line can be attached, so you can give oxygen while ventilating. Room air is 21% oxygen;

by using a pocket mask with oxygen attached and delivering at a rate of 12 L/min, you can give the victim 50% oxygen while doing mouth-to-mask ventilation. The mask is best used along with an oropharyngeal airway to keep the airway open. Hold the mask firmly on the face by placing your thumbs on the side of the mask and grasping the lower jaw with the index, middle, and ring fingers. You should hold the jaw at the angle just below the earlobes; pull upward to pull the airway open. Ventilate through the opening of the mask. It is easier for inexperienced personnel to ventilate well with this device than with the bag-valve mask.

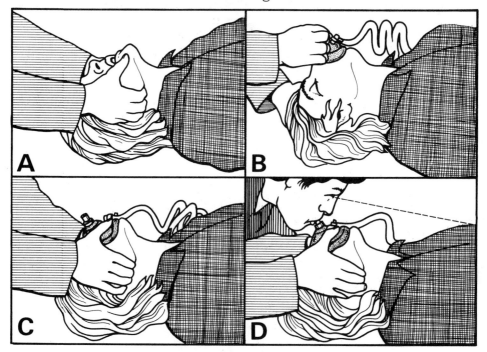

Figure 2-18. Pocket mask.

C. Bag-valve devices: These devices are self-inflating and can deliver room air (21% oxygen) or an oxygen-enriched air mixture to the patient by way of face mask, EGTA, or ET tube. If a face mask is used, it should be used with an oropharyngeal airway to keep the airway open. If oxygen is available, a flow rate of 12 L/min will increase oxygen concentration to about 40%. By the addition of a reservoir bag, the oxygen concentration can be effectively doubled to 80% to 90%. All resuscitation bag-valve devices should have this attached. A disadvantage of the use of bag-valve devices is that the tidal volume is limited by the size of the bag, the size of your hand, and the seal of the mask on the face. The tidal volume is almost always less than with mouth ventilation. This is partially offset by the increased concentration of oxygen that can be delivered with the bag system. Another major disadvantage is that usually two rescuers are needed to adequately ventilate. One must seal the mask on the face while the other squeezes the bag to ventilate.

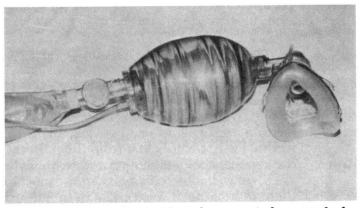

Figure 2-19. Bag-valve mask with reservoir bag attached.

D. Oxygen-powered breathing devices: Manually triggered devices are in general use and operate on compressed oxygen. They attach to a face mask, EGTA, or ET tube. When a button is pushed, high flow oxygen that expands the chest is delivered. You cannot feel lung compliance as accurately with this method as you can with mouth or bag ventilation. The trauma patient often has an injury to his chest, and excessive pressure may cause or worsen a tension pneumothorax. These devices should *not* be used in the trauma victim.

E. Spontaneously breathing patient

1. Many victims who are breathing spontaneously should receive oxygen-enriched air. Examples include those patients with carbon monoxide poisoning, smoke inhalation, chest injuries, head injuries, or shock. There are several methods for accomplishing this:

a. Plastic face mask: This is usually well tolerated, but some patients cannot stand a face mask because they feel they are smothering. If you use a face mask, give oxygen at a rate of 12 L/min, which will deliver about 50% oxygen.

b. Face mask with reservoir bag (nonrebreathing mask): This mask has a reservoir bag attached that acts like the reservoir bag on the bag-valve mask—it essentially doubles the concentration of oxygen (80–90%) to the victim. They are not commonly seen in ambulances but should be carried.

    c. Nasal cannulas: These are usually well tolerated by everyone. When set at an oxygen rate of 6 L/min, they will deliver 25% to 40% oxygen.

    d. There are other, more sophisticated mask systems available, but limited room in the rescue vehicle dictates that equipment should be kept as simple as possible.

2. General rules on administration of oxygen to trauma victims:

    a. Never withhold oxygen from any patient who is short of breath, has a head injury, or is in shock.

    b. Restlessness is a sign of hypoxia; give a restless patient oxygen and look for a cause of shock.

    c. Trauma victims who have chronic lung disease are much more likely to need oxygen than the average victim. Do not withhold it from them. Because of the danger that they may forget to breathe while on oxygen, you should remain in attendance to remind them to breathe or assist them in breathing. Use the same oxygen flow rates (6 L/min nasal cannula, 12 L/min everything else) as for other victims. The old rule about only giving low flow oxygen to chronic lung disease patients comes from hospital experience where people often go for hours without being seen by an attendant. This does not hold true in the prehospital setting where you are constantly monitoring the patient. The flow rate can be adjusted downward after the patient gets to the hospital and arterial blood gases are checked.

    d. Trauma victims with a respiratory rate less than eight per minute are hypoventilating and need oxygen and assistance.

    e. Trauma victims with a respiratory rate greater than 25 per minute may have acidosis and/or hypoxia or may be hyperventilating from excitement. There is no way to be sure in the prehospital setting if one of these exists, so give all of these people oxygen.

    f. Oxygen flow rates must be kept simple if you are to remember them in the field. A setting of 12 L/min will work best with any device (face mask, bag-valve mask) except nasal cannulas. Anything over 6 L/min is wasted when using nasal cannulas, but a setting of 12 L/min will cause no harm. If you cannot remember the setting, the best rule is to give everyone 12 L/min. Venturi masks use special oxygen settings but are not used in the field, so they are of no concern in the prehospital setting.

Chapter 3

Chest Trauma

Anatomy

The thorax is a bony cage that encloses the following:

1. Heart
2. Lungs
3. Aorta
4. Superior and inferior vena cava
5. Trachea and bronchi
6. Esophagus
7. Diaphragm
8. Spinal cord

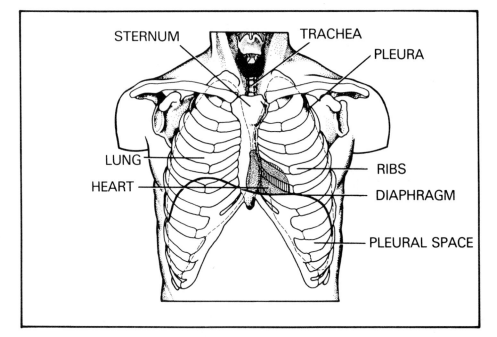

Figure 3-1. Thorax.

Also lying within the bounds of the rib cage are the

1. Kidneys
2. Spleen
3. Liver
4. Pancreas
5. Stomach

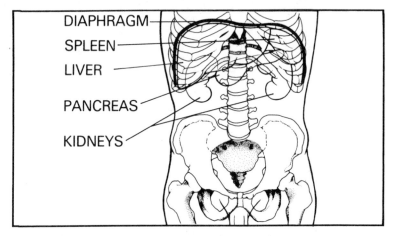

Figure 3-2. Intrathoracic abdomen.

Thus, trauma to the body in the area covered by the rib cage can injure any one or several of the structures listed. Here again, you must be alert to the history and the scene of the accident in order to think of mechanisms of injury. Then a careful, systematic evaluation, keeping in mind the possible injuries, must be made.

Example: A deceleration injury in which a car struck a tree and the driver hit the steering wheel should make you immediately think of the following:

1. Pneumothorax, hemothorax, or tension pneumothorax
2. Rib fractures
3. Sternal fracture
4. Myocardial contusion
5. Cardiac tamponade
6. Thoracic aorta tear
7. Flail chest
8. Spinal cord injury

You must keep priorities in mind as you evaluate the chest since several of the injuries cannot be stabilized in the field and require "load and go" treatment.

In this section we will consider primarily the injuries to the chest and structures above the diaphragm. Those structures in the intrathoracic abdomen will be covered in the section on abdominal injuries.

Pathophysiology

Since there are so many systems involved, pathophysiology will be discussed with each specific injury.

When you are evaluating a victim, always think of the most dangerous injuries first so as to give your patient the greatest chance for survival. If you do a great job splinting an ankle but your patient dies of an airway obstruction, you will never develop the reputation of a lifesaver.

I. **Injuries Capable of Producing Death Within a Few Moments**
    A. Airway obstruction
        1. Evaluation of the airway is always the first priority in evaluating any patient. You must look, listen, and feel for movement of air.
        2. If the victim is making respiratory effort but no air is moving or if he is making no respiratory effort, the airway must be opened immediately. This has already been covered in the section on airway management. Do not forget to stabilize the cervical spine while gaining control of the airway.
    B. Open pneumothorax (sucking chest wound)
        1. Pathophysiology: Normally, the chest expands and the diaphragm contracts, causing a negative pressure inside the chest. Air rushes in through the upper airway and trachea and expands the lungs. When the diaphragm and chest relax, a positive pressure is formed that forces the air back out the same route. If the chest sustains a penetrating injury (e.g., knife or missile) large enough to remain open, air will enter and exit the chest with the change in intrathoracic pressure; however, this air will

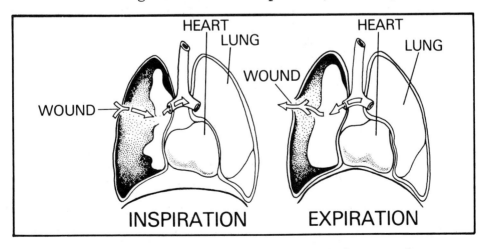

Figure 3-3. Open pneumothorax—sucking chest wound.

only enter the pleural space (causing the lung to collapse). It will not enter the lung and therefore will not contribute to oxygenation of the blood. Air will follow the path of least resistance, so if the opening is larger than the glottic opening, more air will enter the pleural space than the lungs. In other words, the movement of the ribs and diaphragm will be unable to form enough negative pressure to ventilate the lungs, and the victim will smother as surely as if he had an airway obstruction.

2. Diagnosis of sucking chest wound: There is generally no difficulty with this diagnosis. The patient will have sustained some sort of penetrating trauma to the chest, he will have trouble moving air even though his airway is open, and, generally, he will have another opening in the chest that you can both see and hear.

3. Treatment of sucking chest wound:

   a. Close the wound: This can be done with anything that will seal the wound. Have the patient exhale just before you seal the opening. A gel defibrillator pad (Littman, 3M) works best because it will stick to wet or dry skin. Petrolatum gauze or Saran ™ wrap also works well. A more sophisticated dressing can be made by cutting the tip out of a condom and taping the base of the condom over the opening. This will

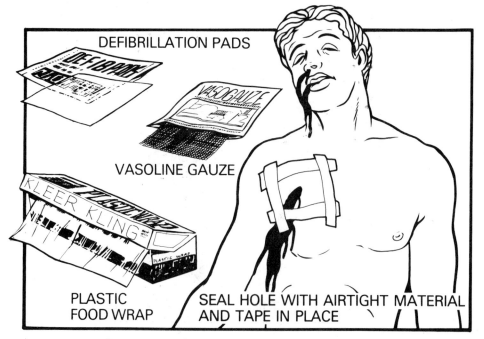

Figure 3-4. Treatment of sucking chest wound.

keep air from entering the chest but will allow air to exit, thus preventing any chance of a tension pneumothorax. For larger wounds, a thin rubber glove with the tip of a finger cut off can be used in the same manner. However, time is so important in this situation that the simpler procedure (defibrillator pad or Saran wrap) is better. You must remain alert to the possibility of a tension pneumothorax developing after you seal the opening. If the patient develops signs of tension pneumothorax, remove the seal momentarily to allow pressure to escape.

b. Give oxygen.

c. If there is *no danger* of spinal injury (stab wound only), you may transport the victim on the affected side. This allows the uninjured lung to function best. If there is any danger of spinal injury, the victim must be transported supine on a spine board with neck stabilized.

d. Notify Medical Control: They should have you start an IV with Ringer's lactate.

C. Tension pneumothorax
   1. Pathophysiology: If only a small amount of air enters the chest, as usually happens with a bullet or stab wound, the lung on the affected side will collapse to a degree equal

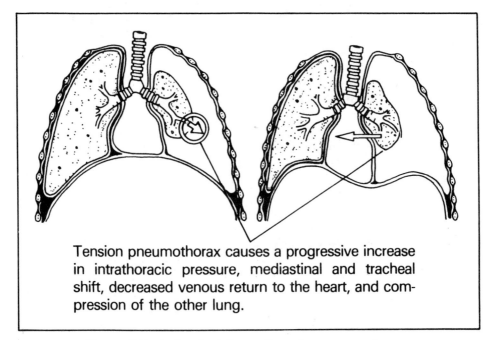

Tension pneumothorax causes a progressive increase in intrathoracic pressure, mediastinal and tracheal shift, decreased venous return to the heart, and compression of the other lung.

Figure 3-5. Pathophysiology of tension pneumothorax.

to the amount of air entering. Young people without preexisting lung disease can tolerate this injury with no difficulty. If the injury is more severe so that major injury to the lung tissue or bronchus is present, air may continue to leak into the pleural space but cannot get out so the lung on the affected side completely collapses and then begins to push the heart and mediastinum across onto the good lung. This causes two problems:
   a.   The good lung is compressed so ventilation is almost impossible.
   b.   The pressure on the mediastinum interferes with the return of the blood to the heart so circulation decreases.

Thus, the victim becomes rapidly hypoxic from lack of ventilation and shocky from hypoxia and decreased cardiac output. Death occurs rapidly once the patient reaches this condition.

2.   Diagnosis of tension pneumothorax:
   a.   There will be a history of penetrating wound to the chest or a deceleration injury (motor vehicle accident or fall) that may have produced a tear of the bronchus or lung. Remember, a penetration wound is not necessary to develop a tension pneumothorax.
   b.   Physical findings: The patient will be in respiratory distress and will appear cyanotic and shocky. He will move air poorly or not at all even with his airway open. Neck veins usually will be distended, the trachea usually will be deviated away from the side of the injury (look at the sternal notch to evaluate), and breath sounds will be absent or decreased on the affected side. The affected side will be hyperresonant to percussion.

3.   Treatment of tension pneumothorax: This injury cannot be stabilized in the field. You must immediately notify your Medical Control physician and prepare to load and go. This patient is dying of hypoxia, so give him oxygen at a wide open rate. If the situation is desperate, you may be asked to decompress the tension pneumothorax by needle aspiration. This is done by inserting a large bore needle in the fifth interspace in the midaxillary line and allowing the air to escape. This converts a tension pneumothorax to a simple pneumothorax. Most people can tolerate a simple pneumothorax without difficulty. The procedure of needle aspiration of the chest will be taught in a skill station.

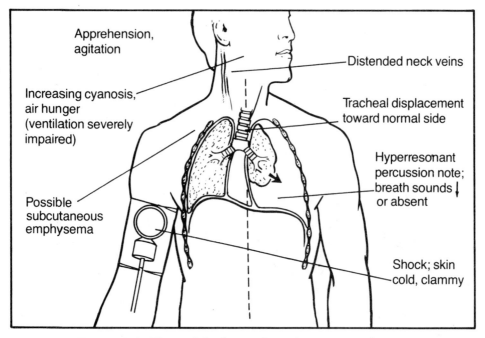

Apprehension, agitation

Increasing cyanosis, air hunger (ventilation severely impaired)

Possible subcutaneous emphysema

Distended neck veins

Tracheal displacement toward normal side

Hyperresonant percussion note; breath sounds ↓ or absent

Shock; skin cold, clammy

Figure 3-6. Physical findings of tension pneumothorax.

D. Flail chest
    1. Pathophysiology: The chest is made up of a series of ribs, each of which connects with the sternum and vertebral column to form a circle. If a fracture occurs in one place in one or more ribs, the chest remains stable and the thorax can expand and contract normally. However, if more than one adjacent rib is fractured in more than one place, the section becomes unstable and normal respiration cannot occur. This unstable section will respond to changes in pressure in the chest just as air does. When the rest of the chest expands, creating a negative intrathoracic pressure, the flail segment will suck in. When the rest of the chest relaxes, creating positive pressure in the chest, the flail section will be pushed out. This motion of the flail segment is "paradoxical" or opposite to the rest of the chest wall. It requires great force to break multiple ribs in multiple places, so there is usually severe contusion of the underlying lung. There may also be associated pneumothorax or hemothorax or both. Depending on the size of the flail segment, there may be severe difficulty with ventilation. Air may actually be sucked back and forth between the two lungs rather than

in and out through the trachea, which causes rapid hypoxia. Depending on the degree of injury to the underlying lung, there may be hypoxia from this also. There is often a myocardial contusion associated with this injury, especially if it involves the anterior chest.

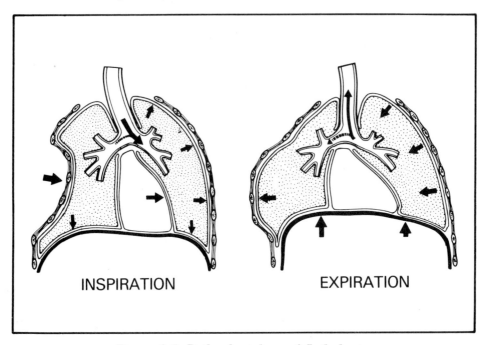

INSPIRATION   EXPIRATION

Figure 3-7. Pathophysiology of flail chest.

2. Diagnosis of flail chest: There is almost always a history of chest trauma from a motor vehicle accident or fall. The victim will usually be moving air poorly in spite of an open airway. Inspection of the chest reveals an unstable section of thorax that moves in a paradoxical manner with respiration. Frequently, other injuries are present, and the patient may be in shock from associated injuries, hypoxia, or myocardial contusion.

3. Treatment of flail chest:

    a. Since the problem is poor ventilation, the first treatment is oxygen at high flow. The next priority is stabilizing the flail segment to improve ventilation. This can be done initially by stabilizing the segment with your hand and then strapping a sandbag or small cushion to the chest over the flail segment. Remember to stabilize the spine and to monitor the heart, and be alert to development of simple pneumothorax or tension pneumothorax. Since this patient usually

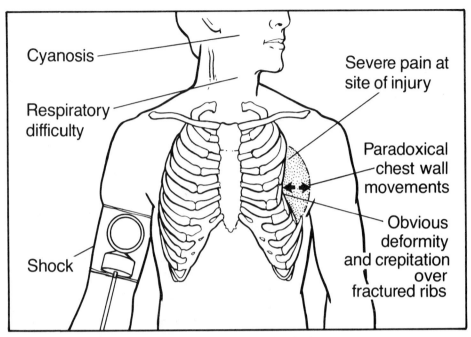

Figure 3-8. Physical findings of flail chest.

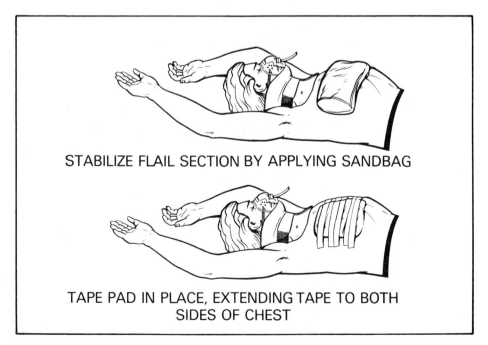

STABILIZE FLAIL SECTION BY APPLYING SANDBAG

TAPE PAD IN PLACE, EXTENDING TAPE TO BOTH SIDES OF CHEST

Figure 3-9. Treatment of flail chest.

has multiple injuries, you may have to treat shock with MAST or intravenous fluids. Remember that unless shock is present, fluids should be limited because excess fluids in the presence of massive lung contusion can lead to pulmonary edema and respiratory failure.

b. Many authors advocate turning the victim onto his affected side to stabilize the chest. Because of the danger of spinal injury in this victim, he should not be transported on his side but rather supine on a spine board with his neck stabilized.

E. Massive hemothorax: The first four injuries discussed have as their primary symptom ventilatory difficulty. The next three (hemothorax, myocardial contusion, and pericardial tamponade) will present themselves primarily with problems in circulation.

1. Pathophysiology: Injuries to lung tissue usually do not cause excessive bleeding because circulation through the lung is under low pressure compared with the rest of the body, and lung tissue is rich in blood clotting factors so injuries tend to seal themselves rapidly. Massive bleeding into the chest is usually caused by an injury to the heart or one of the major intrathoracic blood vessels. Hemothorax may be associated with pneumothorax and may even, although rarely, be a tension hemopneumothorax.

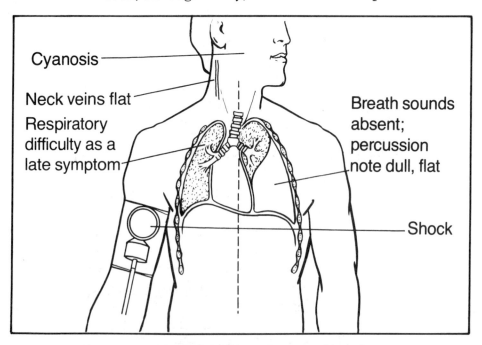

Figure 3-10. Physical findings of massive hemothorax.

2. Diagnosis of massive hemothorax: Instead of acute ventilatory difficulty as seen with pneumothorax, hemothorax presents as shock first and then ventilation problems later. Since the patient is hypovolemic, his neck veins will be flat and he will have dullness to percussion on the affected side.

Comparison of Tension Pneumothorax and Hemothorax

	Tension Pneumothorax	Hemothorax
Primary presenting symptom	Difficulty breathing, then shock	Shock, then difficulty breathing
Neck veins	Distended	Flat
Breath sounds	Decreased or absent on side of injury	Decreased or absent on side of injury
Percussion of chest	Hyperresonant	Dull
Tracheal deviation away from the side of the injury	Present	Usually not present

3. Treatment of massive hemothorax: After your initial evaluation and treatment, you must treat the underlying problem of hemothorax, which is hypovolemic shock. Treatment includes MAST, two large IVs with Ringer's lactate at a rapid rate, and high flow oxygen (remember that shock is a hypoxic state). *Rapid transport* to an emergency facility capable of chest surgery must follow. *You should notify Medical Control early for orders and so that arrangements can be made to have a thoracic surgeon available when you arrive.* Massive hemothorax (especially from penetrating wounds to the chest) is the classic "scoop and run" situation. *All* advanced life support (ALS) procedures should be done *during* transport, *not* at the scene.

F. Myocardial contusion
   1. Pathophysiology: The heart lies just behind the sternum and anterior ribs. Any blunt trauma to the anterior chest transmits force to the heart muscle. Bruising of the heart is essentially the same type injury as a heart attack and shows up with the same symptoms: pain, dysrhythmias, and cardiogenic shock.
   2. Diagnosis of myocardial contusion: You must have a high index of suspicion in any blunt trauma to the anterior chest. Approximately 10% of steering wheel injuries reportedly cause myocardial contusion. In all cases of blunt anterior chest trauma, you should monitor the heart if

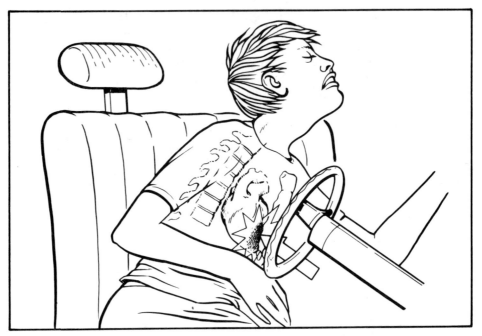

Figure 3-11. Pathophysiology of myocardial contusion.

possible. As stated above, the symptoms are the same as
for a myocardial infarction.

3. Treatment of myocardial contusion: Treatment is the
    same as for chest pain possibly due to myocardial infarc-
    tion. Monitor the heart, give oxygen, start an IV so that
    antidysrhythmic drugs may be given if necessary.

G. Cardiac tamponade

1. Pathophysiology: The pericardium is a fibrous membrane
    that encloses the heart. It will not distend rapidly, so if
    blood collects rapidly between the pericardium and the
    heart, pressure will be applied to the heart muscle,
    squeezing it until the chambers of the heart are so small
    that not enough blood can be pumped to serve the body.
    (Bleeding into the pericardium can be caused by pene-
    trating injuries or blunt trauma to the heart). As the pres-
    sure rises, neck veins distend. The heart sounds become
    muffled because the heart is surrounded by a layer of
    blood and the pulse pressure narrows because the stroke
    volume is decreasing.

2. Diagnosis of cardiac tamponade: The patient will have a
    history of blunt or penetrating trauma to the chest. He
    will be in shock with distended neck veins, yet there will
    be bilateral breath sounds and the trachea will not be
    deviated. The pulse pressure will be decreased (but this

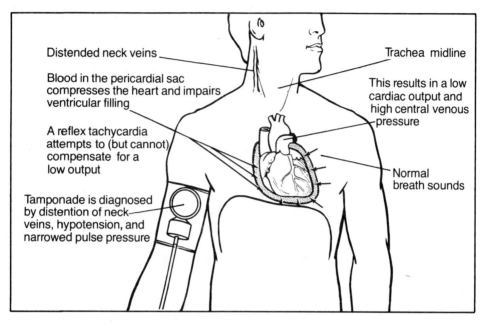

Distended neck veins

Blood in the pericardial sac compresses the heart and impairs ventricular filling

A reflex tachycardia attempts to (but cannot) compensate for a low output

Tamponade is diagnosed by distention of neck veins, hypotension, and narrowed pulse pressure

Trachea midline

This results in a low cardiac output and high central venous pressure

Normal breath sounds

Figure 3-12. Pathophysiology and physical findings of cardiac tamponade.

occurs with all shock), and the heart sounds will be muffled (this occurs in all shock also). Essentially, you must suspect this injury in all patients with chest trauma and differentiate it from tension pneumothorax.

3. Treatment of cardiac tamponade: This is an injury that is rapidly fatal and yet cannot be treated in the field. You must load and go. You can give high flow oxygen and apply MAST, which may increase the venous pressure enough to increase cardiac filling and cardiac output. Remember the rules for initial assessment and treatment, and stabilize the spine when there is blunt trauma deceleration injury.

II. **Other Chest Injuries**
These are mentioned separately because they are either generally not fatal or not treatable in the field.

A. Aortic disruption: This is the most common cause of sudden death in an automobile accident or fall from a height. The aorta tears in the arch, and the patient bleeds to death within a few moments. Ninety percent of these patients die on the spot. Ten percent will have an incomplete tear that does not blow out until later, and they can be saved if the diagnosis is made in the emergency department. You cannot make this diagnosis in the field, and even if you were able to, there is nothing you could do about it.

B. Diaphragmatic hernia: In deceleration injuries where blunt trauma to the abdomen (seat belt injury) occurs, the diaphragm may tear and the contents of the abdomen may be forced up into the chest. This usually presents with ventilatory symptoms much like a pneumothorax and is treated with oxygen and respiratory assistance.

C. Simple pneumothorax: Blunt or penetrating trauma to the chest may cause this; fractured ribs are the main cause in blunt trauma. Most patients with normal lung function can tolerate even a complete pneumothorax on one side. Symptoms, if present, will be related to ventilation. Oxygen is generally all that is required until the patient reaches the hospital. You must continuously monitor the patient to be sure a tension pneumothorax does not develop.

D. Simple rib fractures: This is the most common injury to the chest. It is usually caused by blunt trauma and generally presents as pain with breathing. Pneumothorax may frequently be associated with this injury. No treatment is needed other than oxygen if the patient is short of breath. Be alert to the possible development of pneumothorax or hemothorax, and observe the patient to be sure a flail segment is not present.

E. Sternum fractures: Blunt trauma to the anterior chest may break the sternum. You can usually diagnose this by palpation. Expect myocardial contusion in these patients. Always monitor their cardiac rhythm if possible.

III. **Axioms on Chest Trauma**

A. Do not forget the "ABCs."

B. Call Medical Control early; many of these patients require rapid transport to the emergency department. Your Medical Control physician will help you decide which patients you need to "scoop and swoop."

C. Do not forget the spine.

D. Gunshot wounds to the chest may produce shock by these means:
1. Massive hemothorax
2. Pericardial tamponade
3. Tension pneumothorax
4. Injury to the spine with spinal shock (do not forget to record your brief neurological examination)

E. Assume that trauma patients in shock with no external bleeding have internal bleeding until proven otherwise. Remember to check for tension pneumothorax and cardiac tamponade also.

Chapter 4

Shock

Shock is a state of inadequate tissue perfusion. In other words, not enough oxygen and nutrients are being delivered to the cells to keep them alive.

Normal tissue perfusion requires four intact mechanisms:

1. Functioning pump: the heart
2. Adequate volume of fluid: the blood and plasma
3. Adequate air exchange to get oxygen in the blood
4. Intact vascular system to deliver the oxygen in the blood

A failure of any one of these components can lead to the clinical state of shock.

In the trauma victim, especially in the early stages, the most common cause of shock is blood loss or hemorrhage. Because this course is concerned with trauma, this section on shock will be essentially limited to hemorrhagic (hypovolemic) shock.

Hemorrhagic shock is a clinical syndrome in which there is insufficient blood flow to supply oxygen to the body. It is caused by an injury to the vascular system with a resulting loss of a sufficient amount of blood to compromise tissue perfusion. Burn shock is the same except it is plasma that is lost instead of whole blood.

Pathophysiology of Hemorrhagic Shock

As the blood volume decreases, the amount of blood returning to the heart decreases, which causes the amount of blood pumped to decrease, and the systolic blood pressure begins to fall. Receptors in the aorta and great vessels then signal the release of catecholamines (epinephrine and norepinephrine) which results in peripheral vasoconstriction, increased heart rate, and increased strength of contraction. The effect of this is a shunting of blood from the skin to the vital organs, an increase in the diastolic blood pressure (thus narrowing the pulse pressure: $\frac{\downarrow \text{systolic}}{\uparrow \text{diastolic}} = \downarrow$ pulse pressure), and an increase in myocardial oxygen consumption. This will maintain normal perfusion for awhile, but if blood loss continues, the pressure will eventually fall to the point of inadequate perfusion. At this point, since not enough oxygen is present, anaerobic metabolism begins with resulting acidosis from production of lactic and pyruvic acid. As acidosis becomes more and more severe, there is eventual loss of response to catecholamines. This results in peripheral vasodilatation and marked decrease in circulatory blood volume, leading finally to ventricular fibrillation and death.

Symptoms of Hemorrhagic Shock

The symptoms of hemorrhagic shock reflect the basic physiologic mechanisms:

1. Hypotension (blood pressure of 100 systolic or less): loss of blood volume
2. Pallor: vasoconstriction secondary to catecholamine release
3. Tachycardia (greater than 100/min): cardiac response to catecholamines
4. Confusion or combativeness: decreased cerebral perfusion
5. Tachypnea (greater than 24/min): hypoxia, acidosis
6. Weakness: hypoxia, acidosis
7. Thirst: hypovolemia
8. Diaphoresis: catecholamine release

Many preventable deaths occur in children and young adult trauma victims because their vigorous vasomotor response to hemorrhage enables them to maintain a normal blood pressure and sensorium until they suddenly have a precipitous decrease in blood pressure, followed by an unconsciousness often associated with vomiting and aspiration.

Classification of Hemorrhage

The average adult has about five liters of circulating blood volume. *(10 pts) = 1 UNIT* As this volume is lost, he goes through several stages of clinical signs. The treatment of hemorrhage is to stop the bleeding and then replace the loss. In class I and class II hemorrhage, only fluid is needed, but in class III and class IV hemorrhage, fluids *and blood* must be used. Since blood is generally not available in the field, you will be using a "crystalloid" solution of either Ringer's lactate or normal saline. Ringer's lactate is considered the superior resuscitation fluid since it is most nearly physiologic (closely approximates body fluid) and the lactate is converted to bicarbonate in the liver, thus helping combat the acidosis. [Fluid has to be replaced on a ratio of 3 cc of fluid for every 1 cc of blood lost.] This is because the crystalloid solution leaks through the walls of the vessels and only one third remains as circulating volume; the rest collects in the tissue.

Class I Hemorrhage (Mild)

This represents a loss of 15% or less (750 cc or 1.5 units of blood) of the circulating blood volume. There are no clinical signs other than perhaps a slight increase in pulse. Treatment is 2 to 2.5 liters Ringer's lactate.

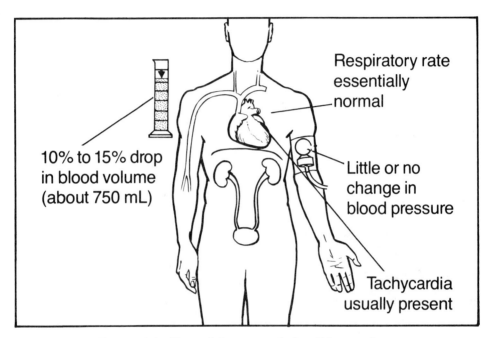

Respiratory rate essentially normal

10% to 15% drop in blood volume (about 750 mL)

Little or no change in blood pressure

Tachycardia usually present

Figure 4-1. Clinical features of class I hemorrhage.

Class II Hemorrhage (Moderate)

This represents a loss of 20% to 25% of circulating blood volume. This is 1,000 cc to 1,250 cc or 2 to 2.5 units of blood, which is considered a major hemorrhage. Clinical signs and symptoms include tachycardia with a pulse rate of 120 or more and tachypnea with a respiratory rate of 24 or more. There will be a drop in the systolic and a rise in the diastolic blood pressure. Along with these, there will probably be weakness, pallor, and thirst. There will be no decrease in urinary output, although this is a value that cannot be measured in the field. A capillary blanch test and tilt test will be positive. Treatment consists of 3 to 4 liters Ringer's lactate IV.

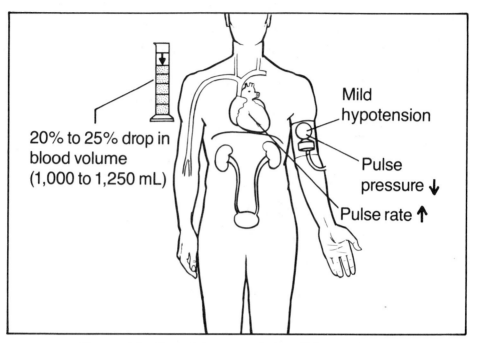

Figure 4-2. Clinical features of class II hemorrhage.

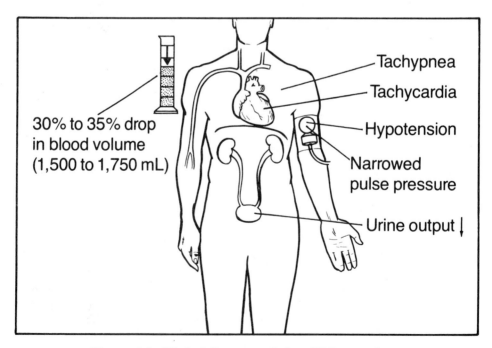

Figure 4-3. Clinical features of class III hemorrhage.

Class III Hemorrhage (Severe)

This represents a loss of 30% to 35% of circulating blood volume. This is 1,500 cc to 1,800 cc or 3 to 3.5 units of blood. The clinical signs are the same as for class II hemorrhage except the blood pressure is obviously low and urinary output is now decreased. Treatment includes volume replacement with a combination of fluids and whole blood.

Class IV Hemorrhage (Catastrophic)

This represents a loss of 40% to 50% of the blood volume. This is 2,000 cc to 2,500 cc or 4 to 5 units of blood. The victim is generally unresponsive with no obtainable blood pressure or pulse. Treatment consists of a combination of fluids, whole blood, and cardiopulmonary resuscitation.

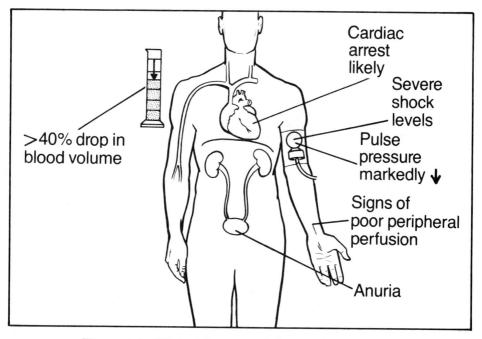

Figure 4-4. Clinical features of class IV hemorrhage.

There are three things to remember when you encounter shock:

1. It is difficult to clinically distinguish between class II and class III hemorrhage in the field.
2. Young people may lose more than 30% of their blood volume before they have a drop in blood pressure.
3. It is easy to underestimate the severity of blood loss until it is too late.

Tests for Early Shock

Capillary Blanch Test

This is an early test for class II hemorrhage. Press on the victim's fingernail or the palm of his hand. The test is positive if the blanched area lasts longer than 2 seconds.

Tilt Test

This is only for use in the patient with no danger of spinal cord injury. Sit the patient upright; the test is positive if he has an increase in his heart rate of greater than 10 beats per minute or a decrease in his systolic blood pressure of 10 mm Hg or more.

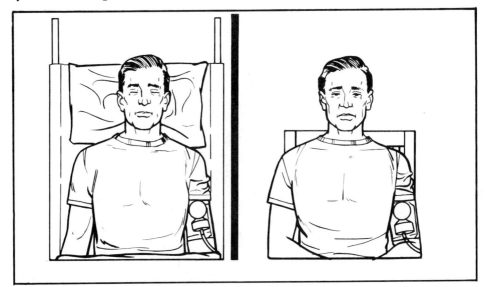

Figure 4-5. Tilt test. The victim is probably in early shock if pulse ↑ 10 beats / min or blood pressure ↓ 10 mm Hg. Do not use this test if there is any danger of spinal injury.

Axioms on Shock

1. Hypotension, tachycardia, and pallor indicate bleeding into the chest or abdomen if no obvious external injuries are present.
2. Hypotension is rarely due to head injury; look elsewhere for blood loss.

3. The degree of head injury cannot be accurately assessed in the presence of deep shock.
4. The smell of alcohol should not influence your assessment in the emergency situation.
5. If the patient is confused, think of head injury or shock before attributing the confusion to inebriation.
6. The talking or shouting patient has an adequate airway.

Management of Shock

Begin with the routine treatment priorities:

1. Open the airway and control the cervical spine.
2. Assess breathing and circulation.
3. Stop the bleeding.
4. Treat the shock.

While you are going through your assessment, you should attempt to get a history of the injury to help establish possible mechanisms of injury. It is also important to know about prior medical history and medications when you get this information. Look for a Medic Alert tag.

Secure a good airway; use an ET tube or EGTA if the victim is unconscious (remember to stabilize the cervical spine).

Always give oxygen to patients in shock. This is a syndrome of insufficient tissue oxygenation. Give 6 L/min for nasal cannula. Use 12 L/min for other methods (face mask, EGTA, ET tube).

Stop the bleeding. This is usually done with pressure dressings or direct pressure on the wound; consider air splints or MAST. Use a tourniquet as a last resort. If the patient bleeds through a dressing, *do not remove it;* apply more dressings on top of the first. If you use a tourniquet, note on the run report the time it is applied.

Apply a MAST garment to treat the shock.

Start two large bore IVs, preferably 14 to 16 gauge.

Replace fluids. Remember that a patient who is obviously in hemorrhagic shock needs at least 3 to 4 liters of Ringer's lactate or normal saline.

Keep the patient warm. It takes energy to maintain a normal temperature, and it takes oxygen for energy: the patient in shock has no oxygen to spare.

Monitor vital signs and level of consciousness at least every 15 minutes.

Transport the patient as soon as possible; do not delay for extended attempts at starting an IV. Get the MAST on and move.

Military Anti-Shock Trousers (MAST)

Principle

No one has proven how MAS Trousers work, but the most likely mechanism is an increase in peripheral resistance by way of circumferential compression. The important thing is that *they do work* to improve blood pressure and cerebral circulation in the hemorrhagic or spinal shock victim. They may also be used to tamponade bleeding and immobilize fractures of the pelvis and lower extremities.

Indications for Use in Trauma

1. Systolic blood pressure less than 80 mm Hg
2. Shock-like symptoms and systolic blood pressure of 100 mm Hg or less
3. Pelvic fracture
4. Fracture of lower extremity
5. Spinal shock
6. Massive abdominal bleeding

Contraindications

1. Pulmonary edema
2. Abdominal injury with protruding viscera (may use leg compartments)
3. Pregnancy (may use leg compartments)

Head injuries do not produce shock. If a patient with a head injury develops symptoms of shock, he probably has hypovolemic shock from internal or external blood loss, or he may have spinal shock. This is not a contraindication to the use of MAST and IV fluids. The use of MAST improves cerebral circulation, decreases cerebral ischemia, and inhibits the development of cerebral edema.

Thoracic injuries also are not a contraindication to the use of MAST. In a situation in which thoracic injuries exist, you should try to raise the systolic blood pressure only to the 100 to 110 mm Hg range.

Technique of Applying and Removing MAST

The technique of applying and removing MAST is covered in the skill station. See page 173.

There are three variations of MAST available:

1. Plain garment with no pressure gauges
2. Garment with one gauge that can be rotated among the three compartments
3. Garment with three gauges, one for each compartment

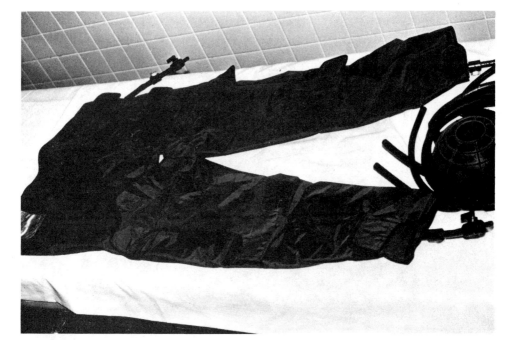

Figure 4-6a. Military anti-shock trousers (MAST)—no pressure gauges.

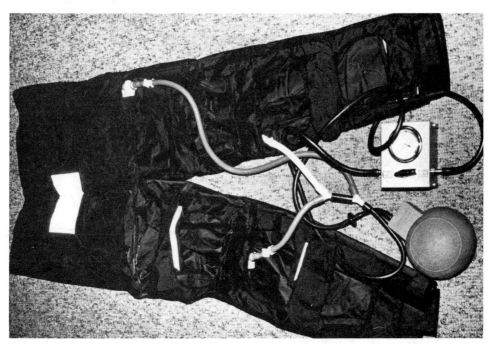

Figure 4-6b. Military anti-shock trousers (MAST)—one pressure gauge.

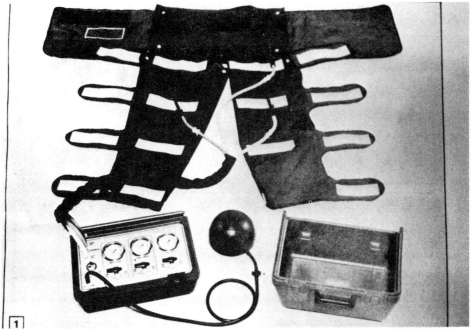

Figure 4-6c. Military anti-shock trousers (MAST)—three pressure gauges.

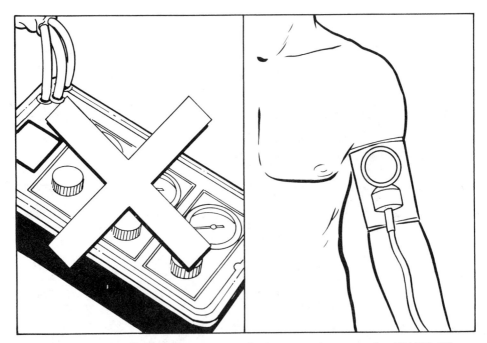

**Figure 4-7. Blood pressure gauge and air pressure gauge for MAST. The
pressure in the victim is what is important!**

For trauma use the plain garment. It is superior since the only gauge you need is a blood pressure cuff on the patient's arm. The danger with having extra gauges is that one tends to become more concerned with the pressure in the suit than the pressure in the patient.

Important Points in the Use of MAST

1. Application of the trousers takes 1 to 2 minutes and immediately improves the patient's condition. Apply the trousers before an IV is attempted unless the patient is trapped or inaccessible. Note the time of inflation on the run report.
2. Application of the trousers will increase the vascular bed in the upper extremities, thereby making venipuncture sites more available.
3. Transportation of a patient in the inflated trousers will minimize displacement of pelvic and other fractures. If a traction splint is required, apply it after the trousers are in place and then inflate the trousers.
4. Once the trousers have been placed on a patient, they should only be removed in a hospital under a physician's direction unless pulmonary edema develops. During removal there must be constant monitoring of the vital signs. A blood pressure drop of 5 mm Hg signals a halt to deflation until more fluid can be replaced. (The greatest danger associated with utilization of the suit is rapid removal by persons unaccustomed to its use.)
5. If the trousers have to be used for an extended length of time (over 1 hour), there will be anaerobic metabolism in the legs. When the trousers are deflated, the lactic acid produced will be returned to the circulation. In this situation two ampules of sodium bicarbonate should be given during the deflation of the trousers to offset this acidosis.

Hemorrhagic Shock: Summary

Hemorrhagic shock is a critical condition that occurs just before death. In the past, treatment has tended to be "too little and too late." However, successful resuscitation is almost always possible if careful, alert evaluation is teamed with aggressive fluid replacement early in the shock syndrome.

Chapter 5

Spinal Cord Trauma

Injuries to the spinal cord occur in over 10% of all multiple trauma patients and in 15% to 20% of all serious head injury patients. The most common victim of a spinal cord injury is a male automobile accident victim who is 18 to 35 years old.

The initial evaluation and stabilization of the spinal injury victim will often determine whether that patient regains normal function or is crippled for life; in no other system evaluation is the rule "first do no harm" more important. Along with the physical and emotional trauma, there are other concerns as well. Today, the estimated cost of lifetime care for a paraplegic is about one million dollars.

The key to preventing further spinal injury is thinking about the possibility of a spinal injury before the patient is moved. You must *always* look for possible mechanisms of spinal injuries. When in doubt, stabilize the spine: the patient will not be harmed by being transported on a spine board with the cervical spine immobilized.

Anatomy of the Spinal Column

The spinal column serves as the main axis of the body. It is flexible to some degree but provides rigidity to the trunk and neck. It is made up of 26 bones (vertebrae) that are divided into five segments:

1. Cervical spine: made up of the seven bones in the neck C_1-7
2. Thoracic spine: made up of the 12 bones in the upper back to which the 12 ribs are attached T_1-12
3. Lumbar spine: made up of the five bones in the lower back L_1-5
4. Sacrum: part of the pelvic girdle
5. Coccyx: the tail bone

Each vertebra consists of a solid body and a vertebral arch through which passes the spinal cord and spinal nerve roots. Thus, the spinal column also serves as a protector of the spinal cord. Each vertebra is separated by an intervertebral disc that serves as a cushion and allows motion in the spine.

59

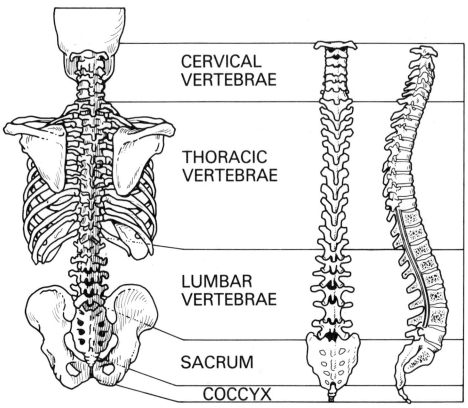

Figure 5-1. Anatomy of spinal column.

CERVICAL VERTEBRAE

THORACIC VERTEBRAE

LUMBAR VERTEBRAE

SACRUM

COCCYX

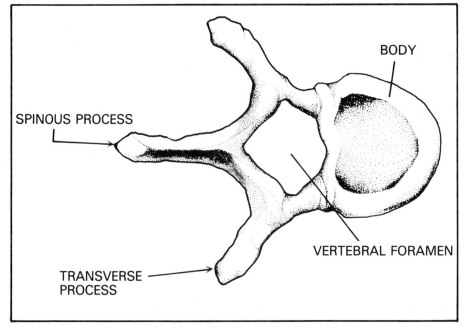

BODY

SPINOUS PROCESS

VERTEBRAL FORAMEN

TRANSVERSE PROCESS

Figure 5-2. Vertebra viewed from above.

The Spinal Cord

The spinal cord is a continuation of the central nervous system outside of the skull. It is like an electrical cable extending down through the vertebral foramen of the spinal column with the nerve roots exiting between every vertebrae. This is a two-way conduction system bringing sensory messages to the brain and sending motor messages to the muscles and organs. If the cord is transected at any point, there is complete loss of motor, sensory, and reflex activity below that area. Thus, an injury to the lumbar area of the cord would cause paralysis of both legs but would not affect the arms. An injury in the neck would cause paralysis of both arms and both legs.

Fractures or dislocations of the spinal column may occur without injury to the spinal cord, but the potential for injury is always present and may become a reality with improper handling. Conversely, injury to the spinal cord may occur without fracture or dislocation of the vertebrae.

Most injuries to the spine and spinal cord occur in the cervical spine because it is relatively unprotected compared with the rest of the spine. It is also poorly supported in most automobile seats. Since it is the stalk on which the head sits, any forces acting upon the head are transmitted to the neck. The magnitude of these forces is often very great and frequently causes fracture or dislocation of the cervical vertebrae, which, in turn, injures the spinal cord that passes through the small intervertebral foramen.

The thoracic spine is well stabilized by the rib cage and is usually well supported in most automobile seats. Thus, it is injured much less often. If an injury does occur to the thoracic spine, there is a high probability of spinal cord injury because the intervertebral foramen is smallest in this region of the spine.

If there is *any* possibility of injury to the spine, treat the patient as if an injury were present.

Causes of Spinal Injury

There are certain situations that should make you think immediately of the danger of spinal injury.

Motor Vehicle Accident

Any sudden deceleration injury can cause flexion or extension injury to the spine. This can happen even when seat belts are worn. All victims of motor vehicle accidents should be assumed to have spinal injuries until proven otherwise.

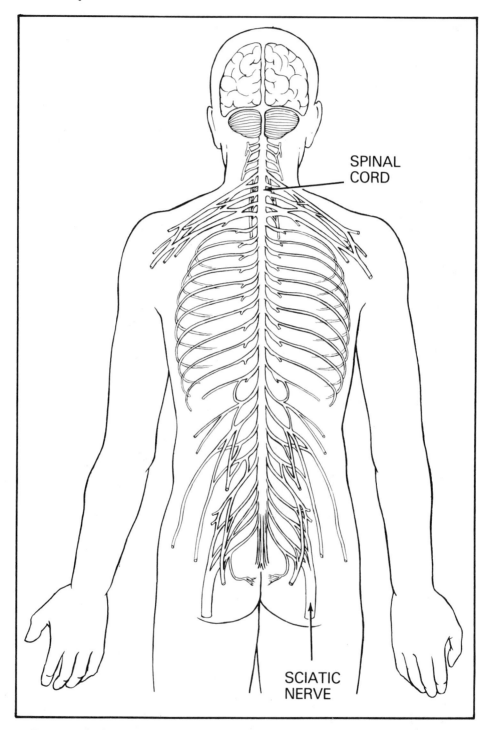

**Figure 5-3. Spinal cord. The spinal cord is a continuation of the central
nervous system outside of the skull.**

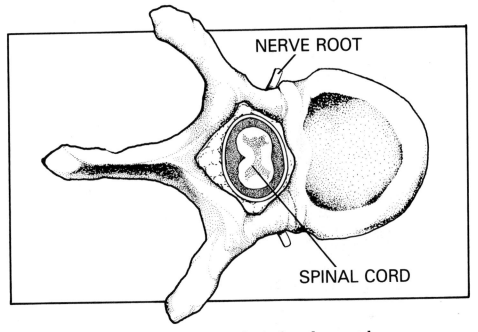

Figure 5-4. Relationship of spinal cord to vertebra.

Fall

The height of the fall and the manner in which the body strikes the ground determines where and what type spinal injury may occur. Remember that there is the possibility of thoracic aortic injury here also.

Diving

This tends to be a flexion injury to the cervical spine. It often occurs in the upper cervical spine (Jefferson fracture) and is a frequent cause of drowning. You must think of this injury if you are called to rescue a drowning victim. The victim's neck must be stabilized immediately if there is a history of diving preceding the rescue.

Athletic Competition

High risk sports include tackle football, surfing, diving, wrestling, gymnastics, and trampoline. Cervical spine fractures are the number one cause of fatal football injuries.

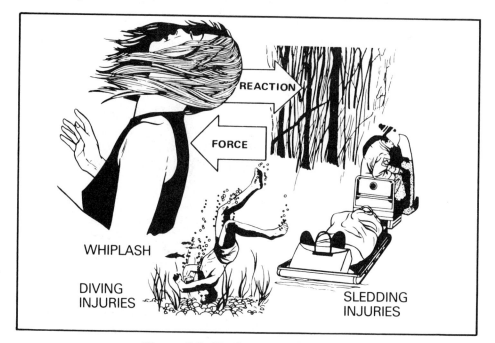

Figure 5-5. Mechanisms of injury.

Penetrating Trauma

Gunshot wounds to the neck, chest, or abdomen may directly penetrate the spinal cord. Knife wounds of the neck or back may penetrate or lacerate the cord.

Electric Shock

Spinal injury may occur from direct electrical injury or by the violent muscle spasm that accompanies electrical shock.

Sudden Twist

Often this is all it takes to cause herniation of a degenerated intervertebral disc into the intervertebral foramen, causing pressure on the spinal cord. You must consider this when there is a history of sudden, severe neck or back pain.

Specific Injuries

The spinal cord may be bruised, compressed, lacerated, or completely transected. The cord does not tolerate compression well—even for short periods of time.

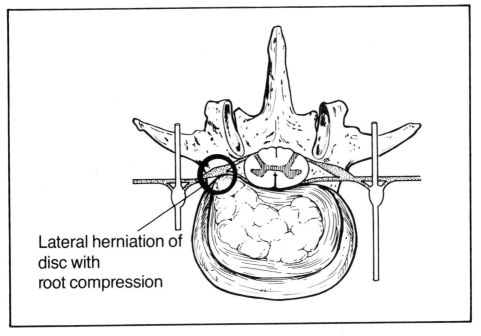

Lateral herniation of
disc with
root compression

Figure 5-6. Herniated intervertebral disc.

The phrenic nerve controls respiration. Its roots come out between the third, fourth, and fifth cervical vertebrae. Injuries to the cord above this level cause respiratory paralysis; most patients with this injury die at the scene. Injuries to the cord below the fifth cervical vertebra but above the thoracic vertebrae cause paralysis of the intercostal muscles, but victims can still breathe with their diaphragms.

A total disruption of the cord causes loss of motor function, sensation, and reflexes below the level of the injury. There can be various degrees of injury to the cord so that one or more functions may be lost but the others remain; thus, you should quickly evaluate motor function and sensation in both hands and both feet.

Whiplash: Cervical Strain

This is the most common injury from a rear end automobile collision. It is a hyperextension injury with tearing and stretching of the anterior neck muscles. A 15-mile-per-hour rear end collision can accelerate the head backward with a force of ten times the pull of gravity.

Spinal Shock: Neurogenic Shock

Spinal shock is caused by loss of the sympathetic control of the capillary bed. Thus, there is a pooling of blood, and the blood pressure

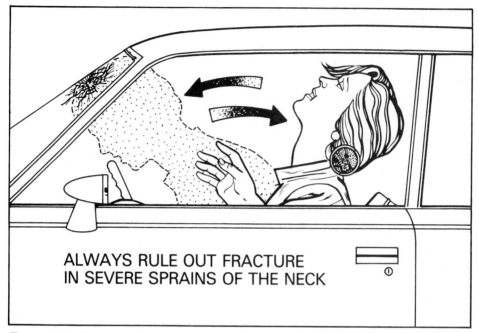

ALWAYS RULE OUT FRACTURE
IN SEVERE SPRAINS OF THE NECK

Figure 5-7. Cervical strain. Severe strain is usually evident from the history of the accident. Hyperextension or hyperflexion is often the mechanism of injury, which may involve either stretching or tearing of ligaments. Symptoms include neck immobility (caused by pain) and spasm of injured muscles.

drops. Since there is no release of catecholamines, there is no pallor or tachycardia. The patient with spinal shock will have a decreased blood pressure, but the pulse will be slow and strong, the skin will be warm and dry, and the patient often will be oriented and alert. Spinal shock responds poorly to fluid replacement but is easily corrected with the application of MAST. It may also be treated with dopamine (Intropin®) or norepinephrine (Levophed®).

Hypothermia

With spinal cord injury there is loss of thermoregulatory mechanisms, so if the patient is not covered, he can experience a rapid loss of body heat with resultant hypothermia.

Central Cord Syndrome

As was mentioned before, injury to the spinal cord *usually* affects everything distal to that area. An injury to the cord in the neck causes weakness or paralysis in the arms, trunk, and legs. However, there is a particular situation in which this is not true. If there is bruising of the center of the spinal cord in the neck, the position of the motor and sensory nerves (arms are more medial—see illustration) will cause weakness or paralysis of the arms without the legs being affected.

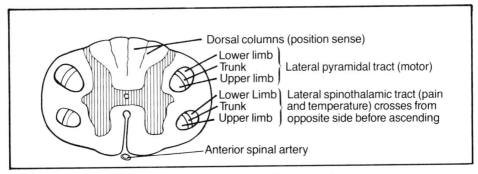

Figure 5-8a. Spinal cord orientation.

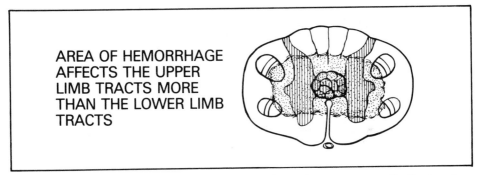

AREA OF HEMORRHAGE AFFECTS THE UPPER LIMB TRACTS MORE THAN THE LOWER LIMB TRACTS

Figure 5-8b. Central cord syndrome. Involves hemorrhage and edema of central cord. On either side of the cord, parts of the three main tracts are involved so that upper limbs are affected more than lower limbs.

Brief Neurological Examination for Possible Spinal Cord Injury

The purpose of this examination is to document loss of sensation and/or motor function. This does not have to be a detailed examination in the field. Parts of the examination obviously cannot be done in the unconscious patient.

I. **Sensory: Conscious Patient**
Ask if he can feel you touch him lightly on each hand and each foot. If he cannot feel light touch, try pin prick. If there is a sensory loss, record the level at which sensation stops; make a mark on the skin of the abdomen or chest with a ball point pen.

II.   **Motor: Conscious or Unconscious Patient**
Ask him to move the fingers of each hand and toes of each foot.
If the patient is unconscious, does he make any spontaneous move-
ment? Does he move in response to pain?

III.   **Reflexes**
This is probably not a useful examination in the field. A total
transection of the cord will cause loss of sensation, motor function,
and reflexes. If any sensation or motor function remains, there is
a chance for recovery.

Priority Plan

Arrival at the Scene

You must make a quick assessment of the overall situation. Quickly
note from the scene the apparent mechanisms of injury.

All victims of motor vehicle accidents should be assumed to have
spinal injury until proven otherwise. All unconscious patients should be
assumed to have spinal injuries as well along with all head or facial
injury patients. Think of spinal injuries in falls, diving accidents, near
drownings, gunshot wounds (of neck, chest, or abdomen), explosions,
and electrocution injuries.

Initial Assessment of the Patient
with Possible Spinal Injury

This begins immediately—even before extrication. Begin with routine
assessment and treatment priorities.

I.   **Secure Airway and Control Cervical Spine**
You must stabilize the spine as you evaluate and secure the
airway. First stabilize the head in a neutral position by holding
steady traction with your hands on either side of the head. If
the victim is unconscious, an airway (EGTA or ET tube) should
be inserted. Remember that the neck must not be extended
when there is a chance of spinal cord injury. If the victim is face
down, one rescuer must hold the neck in a neutral position by
in-line traction while other rescuers log roll the victim onto a
spine board.

II.   **Check Breathing**
A.   As you check the breathing, you should also look at the neck
(for neck vein distention, tracheal injury or deviation, and
tenderness or abnormality of the cervical spine) and then
apply a Philadelphia collar and sandbags or comparable stabilizing apparatus (foam rubber choke collars are not adequate).

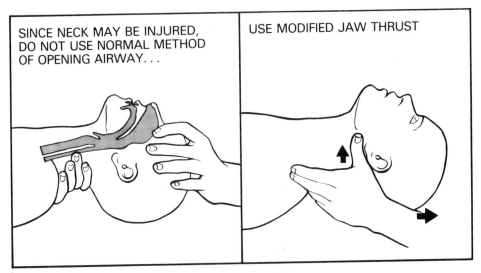

SINCE NECK MAY BE INJURED, DO NOT USE NORMAL METHOD OF OPENING AIRWAY...

USE MODIFIED JAW THRUST

Figure 5-9. Modified jaw thrust.

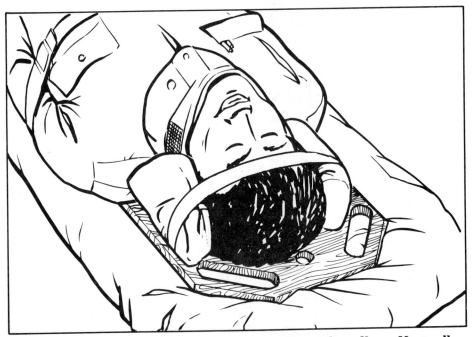

Figure 5-10. Spine board with Philadelphia collar and sandbags. Most collars do not give adequate lateral stabilization—use sandbags also.

B. Control of circulation: If cardiopulmonary resuscitation is required, you must extricate the victim and place him on a firm surface. A spine board is perfect and also protects the thoracic and lumbar spine. Do not forget that drowning victims requiring cardiopulmonary resuscitation often have neck injuries (diving injury); if you extend the neck, you can

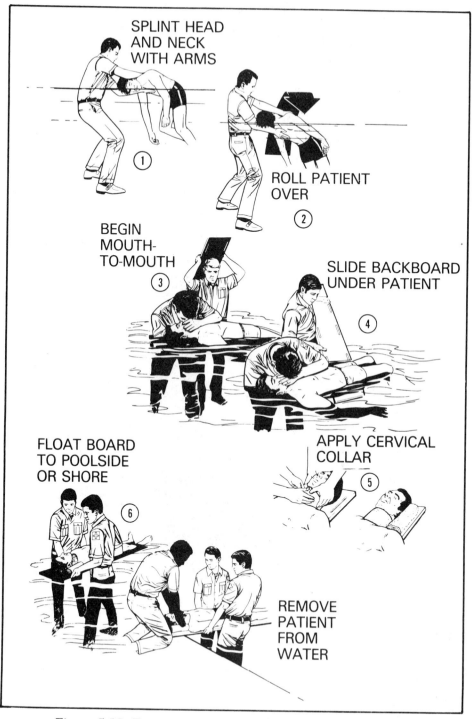

SPLINT HEAD
AND NECK
WITH ARMS

1

ROLL PATIENT
OVER

2

BEGIN
MOUTH-
TO-MOUTH

3

SLIDE BACKBOARD
UNDER PATIENT

4

FLOAT BOARD
TO POOLSIDE
OR SHORE

6

APPLY CERVICAL
COLLAR

5

REMOVE
PATIENT
FROM
WATER

Figure 5-11. Extricating suspected diving accident victim.

cause complete paralysis. Always stabilize the neck if there is any possibility that a diving injury has occurred.

III. **Stop the Bleeding**
IV. **Treat the Shock**
   Observe for the difference between hemorrhagic and spinal shock.
 V. **Perform Neurological Examination**
   As you do the secondary survey, have another teammate splint the fractures. Do your neurological examination now. Include level of consciousness, eye opening, pupils, ability to speak, bilateral movement of fingers and toes, and bilateral sensory examination. If there is a loss of sensation, record and mark the level on the patient.
VI. **Obtain a History of the Injury**
   A.   Personal observation
   B.   Bystanders' observations
   C.   Patient's description
   D.   Important points: Was the patient moved before you arrived? For the paralyzed patient, did he have any movement before you arrived? Were there any changes in his condition before you arrived?
VII. **Contact Medical Control**
VIII. **Transport with Continuous Monitoring**

Tips on Management

1.   If there is an obvious spinal injury with paralysis, be sure to put the MAST on the spine board since the patient may go into spinal shock.
2.   Be sure the patient is securely immobilized on the spine board. A patient with spinal injury is likely to vomit, so he and the board must be able to be rolled to the side to prevent aspiration of vomitus.
3.   It is usually best to remove crash helmets in the field. If it is left in place, the helmet may be removed eventually by someone not trained in the proper procedure. If there is a neck injury, an improper technique during removal of the helmet could cause spinal injury.
4.   Do not allow a patient with possible spinal injuries to sit or stand.
5.   Cover the patient to prevent hypothermia.

Summary

Always be alert to mechanisms that may produce injuries of the spine. When in doubt, immobilize; your first duty is to prevent further injury.

Chapter 6

Head Trauma

About 40% of trauma victims have central nervous system injuries. This group has a death rate twice as high as that of victims with other types of injuries (35% versus 17% overall). As with other injuries, organized systematic evaluation and treatment gives the patient the greatest chance for complete recovery. To understand evaluation and management of head injuries, you must have some knowledge of the basic anatomy and physiology of this area.

Anatomy of the Head

The head (excluding the face and facial structures) is made up of the following:

1. Scalp
2. Skull
3. Fibrous coverings of the brain
4. Brain substance
5. Cerebrospinal fluid
6. Vascular compartments

The skull is like a closed box; the only significant opening is the foramen magnum at the base where the spinal cord exits. The rigid, unyielding nature of the skull is the basis of several injury mechanisms in head trauma.

Pathophysiology of Head Trauma

It is best to think of the brain as being fluid in nature. Most brain injuries are not from direct injury to brain tissue but occur due to the movement of the brain inside the skull. In deceleration injuries the head usually strikes some object, such as the windshield, which causes a sudden stop of the head and skull. Inside the skull, the brain moves forward, impacting first against the original blow and then rebounding and hitting the opposite side of the inner surface of the skull. Injuries

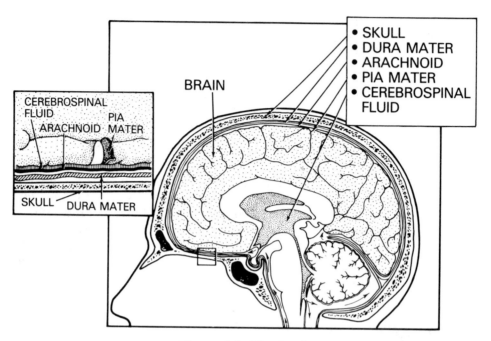

Figure 6-1. The head.

may occur to the brain in the area of the original blow (coup) or on the opposite side (contrecoup). This movement inside the skull causes most of the injuries seen post trauma.

The base of the skull is rough. Movement over this area causes various degrees of injury to the brain substance or blood vessels serving the brain.

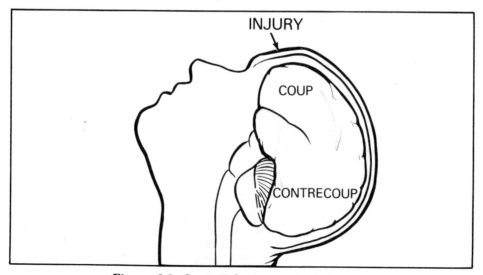

Figure 6-2. Coup and contrecoup injuries.

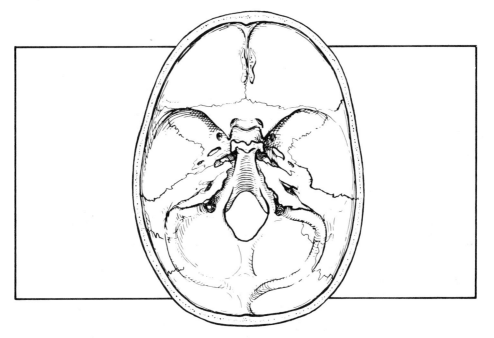

Figure 6-3. Base of skull.

The *initial* response of the bruised brain is swelling. This is from increased blood volume because of vasodilatation and increased cerebral blood flow to the injured areas. The buildup of this extra blood volume exerts pressure on the brain, eventually causing decreased blood flow to the uninjured parts of the brain. The buildup of increased cerebral water (edema fluid) does not occur immediately but develops over the next 24 to 48 hours. This is an important concept in that *early* efforts to decrease the vasodilatation in the injured areas can have a profound effect on the patient's eventual outcome.

The blood level of carbon dioxide (CO_2) has a critical effect on cerebral vessels. The normal blood $PaCO_2$ is 40 mm Hg. Increasing the $PaCO_2$ causes vasodilatation, while decreasing the $PaCO_2$ causes vasoconstriction. If the patient is not ventilated well, there will be even further vasodilatation and an increase in intracerebral pressure. Hyperventilation can decrease the $PaCO_2$ to 25 mm Hg, causing an immediate vasoconstriction of the cerebral vessels. This will help prevent the buildup of blood in the injured areas and allow *better* perfusion of the entire brain. Hyperventilation is a critical point in treatment of head injury. Early in the course of the injury, hyperventilation is more important than the administration of mannitol or Lasix®. Mannitol and Lasix reduce edema fluid by diuresis; edema fluid usually does not develop for several hours, so administration of these drugs can wait until after the victim is in the hospital. Early administration of mannitol may actually be deleterious since it causes some vasodilatation. Any victim who shows signs of increasing intracranial pressure should have immediate hyperventilation.

Head injuries may be the result of bruising of the brain substance with resulting swelling and pressure on the rest of the brain, tearing of blood vessels with resulting bleeding and development of pressure on the brain, or direct penetrating injuries to the brain substance from foreign objects (bullets and knives, for example) or pieces of bone from a skull fracture.

Intracranial Pressure

Inside the skull and fibrous coverings of the brain are the brain tissue, cerebrospinal fluid, and blood. Any increase in the size of one of these must be at the expense of the other two because the skull will not expand. The only part of the system that can "give" is the cerebrospinal fluid, but even if this fluid were "squeezed" out of the skull completely, there would be little extra space. Blood supply cannot be compromised, for the brain tissue must have a good, continuous supply of blood to function. Thus, since none of the components of the brain can be compromised, an injury to or swelling of the brain will precipitate an increase in intracranial pressure.

The pressure of the blood flowing through the brain is called the cerebral perfusion pressure. Its value is obtained by subtracting the intracranial (intracerebral) pressure from the mean arterial blood pressure. If the brain swells or if there is bleeding inside the skull, the intracerebral pressure increases and the perfusion pressure decreases. The body has a protective reflex (Cushing reflex) that works to maintain a constant perfusion pressure: if the intracerebral pressure increases, there will be a concurrent rise in blood pressure to try to maintain

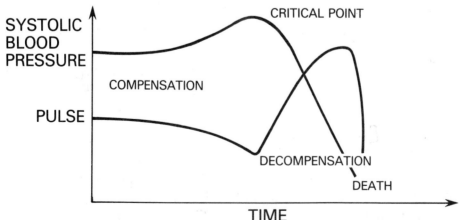

Figure 6-4. Cushing response.

blood flow in the brain. This will continue until a critical point at which time *all* vital signs will decrease and the patient will eventually die.

A very important point to remember here is that head injuries (if there is increased intracranial pressure) tend to cause an *increase* in blood pressure so the presence of shock, which usually causes a *decrease* in blood pressure, in a head injury patient is probably due to bleeding or spinal cord injury. *Head injuries are not necessarily the cause of the shock.* You must therefore look for and treat the cause. Unexplained rises in blood pressure in a head trauma patient may indicate a worsening intracranial injury causing increased intracranial pressure. Falling blood pressure from head trauma occurs only as a terminal event.

Anoxic Brain Injury

Injuries to the brain from lack of oxygen (e.g., cardiac arrest, choking, drowning) affect the brain differently from direct trauma. If the brain goes more than 4 to 6 minutes without oxygen, spasm develops in the small arteries so that if the brain is reperfused, blood will not flow to the cortex, and the patient will die within a day or so from brain failure. This arterial spasm is related to flow of calcium into the arterial muscle cells; complete spasm does not occur for approximately 90 minutes.

It has long been thought that the brain could not be resuscitated after 4 to 6 minutes of anoxia, but with a new class of drug becoming available (the calcium blockers), there is hope of brain recovery if resuscitation is begun sometime during the 90-minute period before complete arterial spasm shuts off all blood flow to the cortex.

Injuries

Scalp Wounds

The scalp is very vascular and can bleed extensively when cut. This can be very important in children who bleed as freely as adults but have much less blood volume to lose. As a general rule, adults with scalp injuries who are in shock usually have their shock caused by some other site of bleeding (often internal). Most bleeding from the scalp is easily controlled with direct pressure.

Skull Injuries

Skull injuries can be linear nondisplaced fractures, depressed skull fractures, and compound skull fractures. There is very little you can do in the field for these except to remember not to put pressure on an obvious depressed skull fracture. Penetrating objects in the skull should be left in place and the victim transported immediately to the emergency room.

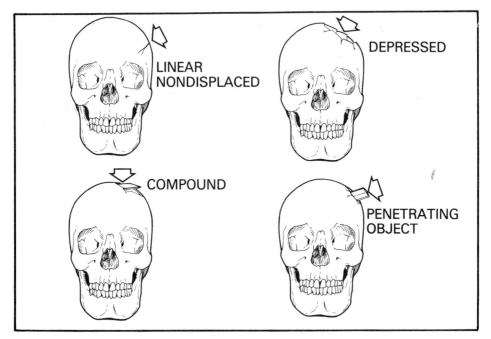

Figure 6-5. Skull fracture—linear nondisplaced, depressed, compound, and penetrating object.

Brain Injuries

There are several types of brain injuries. The following outline briefly discusses some of these.

I. **Concussion**

   A concussion implies no significant injury to the brain itself. There is usually a history of trauma to the head with a variable period of unconsciousness or confusion and then a return to normal consciousness. There may be amnesia from the injury. This amnesia usually extends to some point before the injury so that often the patient will not remember the events leading to the injury. There may be dizziness, headache, or nausea. This patient requires a period of observation; if unconsciousness lasts for 5 minutes or more, usually he should be admitted to the hospital for observation.

II. **Cerebral Contusion**

   A patient with cerebral contusion will have a history of prolonged unconsciousness or serious alteration in his state of consciousness (e.g., will often ask the same question over and over). He may have focal neurological signs. This patient should be admitted for observation.

III. **Intracranial Hemorrhage**

Hemorrhage can occur between the skull and the dura (the fibrous covering of the brain), between the dura and the brain, or in the brain tissue itself.

A. Acute epidural hematoma: This is a rare injury (less than 1% of head injuries) that is usually caused by a tear in the middle meningeal artery. It is often associated with a linear skull fracture in the temporal or parietal region. Because it is arterial bleeding, pressure can rise rapidly so death occurs quickly. Surgical removal of the blood and ligation of the artery often gives excellent recovery, for often the underlying brain tissue is not injured. The symptoms include a history of head trauma with initial loss of consciousness followed by a period during which the patient is conscious and coherent. Later, the patient will lapse into unconsciousness and develop a paralysis on the opposite side from the injury. (There is usually a dilated and fixed pupil on the same side as the injury.) Usually, this is followed rapidly by death. The classic example is the boxer who is knocked unconscious, wakes up, and is

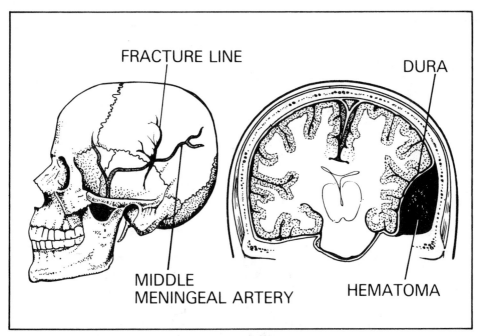

FRACTURE LINE

DURA

MIDDLE MENINGEAL ARTERY

HEMATOMA

Figure 6-6. Acute epidural hematoma. This hemorrhage may follow injury to the extradural arteries. The blood collects between the fibrous dura and the periosteum.

allowed to go home only to be found dead in bed the next morning.

B. Acute subdural hematoma: This is caused by bleeding between the dura and the brain substance and is associated usually with injury to the underlying brain tissue. Because the bleeding is venous, pressure develops more slowly, and often the diagnosis is not made for hours after the injury. The signs and symptoms include headache, fluctuations in the level of consciousness, and hemiparesis. Because of underlying brain tissue injury, prognosis is often poor. Mortality is very high (60% to 90%) in victims who are comatose when found. Recent studies have found that early surgery reduces mortality. The mortality rate for those patients on whom surgery is performed less than 4 hours following the injury is 30%. The mortality rate for surgery performed more than 4 hours after injury is 90%.

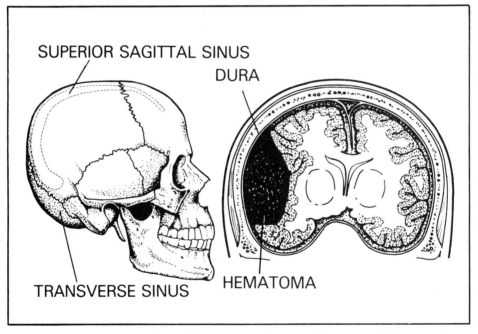

SUPERIOR SAGITTAL SINUS

DURA

TRANSVERSE SINUS   HEMATOMA

Figure 6-7. Acute subdural hematoma. This usually occurs following the rupture of dural vessels (veins). Blood collects and often severely compresses and distorts the brain.

C. Intracerebral hemorrhage: This is bleeding within the brain tissue. It is always associated with penetrating injuries and may be associated with blunt trauma. Surgery is usually not helpful. Symptoms depend upon the amount of injury and areas involved.

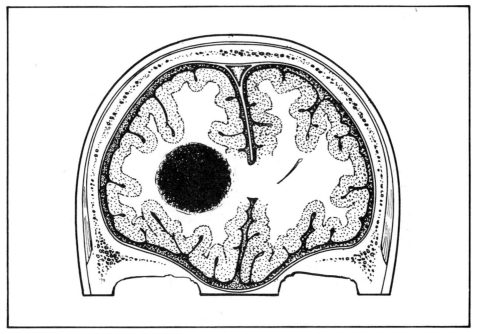

Figure 6-8. Intracerebral hemorrhage.

Evaluation of the Head Trauma Victim

Remember that every trauma victim is initially evaluated in the same sequence:

1. Secure airway and control the cervical spine
2. Assess breathing and circulation
3. Stop the bleeding
4. Treat the shock
5. Evaluate for further injuries, including neurological examination and splinting of fractures
6. Transport with continuous monitoring

Once you have done the first five steps, you begin evaluation of the head injury. It is very important that this be recorded because the treatment is often dictated by changes in the observed signs.

Primary Assessment

I. **Level of Consciousness**
Keep this simple so everyone can understand. The AVPU method is quite adequate.
A Patient is *alert*

V   Patient responds to *vocal* stimuli
P̲   Patient responds to *painful* stimuli
U̲   Patient is *unresponsive*
For a patient in a coma, the Glasgow coma scale is simple and easy to use and has good prognostic value as to eventual outcome. It is included at the end of the chapter.

II.   **Vital Signs**

These are extremely important in following the course of head trauma. They indicate changes in intracranial pressure. You should record vital signs every 5 minutes if possible.

A.   Blood pressure: Increasing intracranial pressure causes an increased blood pressure; remember that other things do as well such as fear, hypertension, and pain.

B.   Pulse: Increasing intracranial pressure causes the pulse to decrease.

C.   Respiration: Increasing intracranial pressure causes the respiratory rate to decrease. There may be several other respiratory patterns depending on the injury. As a terminal event, the patient may show central neurogenic hyperventilation, which is a rapid, noisy respiration. Respiration is affected by so many factors (e.g., fear, hysteria, chest injuries, spinal cord injuries, diabetes) that it is not as useful an indicator as the other signs in monitoring the course of head injury.

Comparison of Vital Signs in Shock and Head Injury

	Shock	Head Injury with Increasing Intracranial Pressure
Blood pressure	↓	↑
Pulse	↑	↓
Respiration	↑	↓
Level of consciousness	↓	↓

Secondary Assessment

All patients with head or facial trauma must be thought of as having cervical spine injuries until proven otherwise. Stabilization of the cervical spine begins with airway and breathing evaluation.

Once the primary survey is completed and recorded, begin with the head and quickly, but carefully, examine for obvious injuries such as lacerations or depressed or open skull fractures. The size of lacerations is often misjudged because of the difficulty of finding them in hair matted with blood. Feel the scalp with your fingers for obvious unstable areas of the skull. If none are present, apply a pressure dressing or hold direct pressure to stop the bleeding.

A basilar skull fracture may be indicated by bleeding from the ear or from the nose, swelling and discoloration behind the ear (Battle's sign), and/or swelling and discoloration around both eyes (raccoon eyes). *LATE SIGNS*

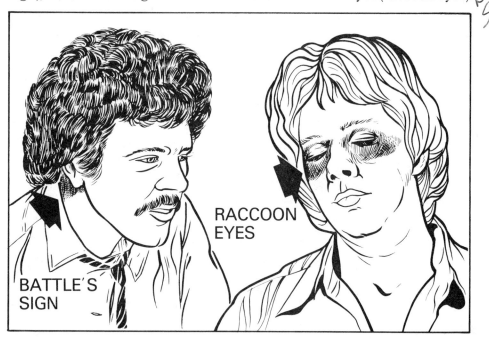

RACCOON EYES

BATTLE'S SIGN

Figure 6-9. Signs of basilar skull fracture—Battle's sign and raccoon eyes.

Pupils

The pupils are controlled by the third cranial nerve. This nerve takes a long course through the skull and is easily compressed by brain swelling, so it may be an early indicator of increasing intracranial pressure. If both pupils are dilated and do not react to light, the patient probably has a brainstem injury and the prognosis is grim. If the pupils are dilated but still react to light, the injury is probably still reversible, so every effort should be made to get the patient quickly to a facility capable of treating a head injury. A unilaterally dilated pupil that remains reactive to light may be the earliest sign of increasing intracranial pressure. The development of a unilaterally dilated pupil while you are observing the pupils is a sign of extreme emergency—in other words, scoop and run!

Fluttering eyelids are often seen with hysteria. Slow lid closure (like a curtain falling) is never seen with hysteria.

If the brainstem is intact, the eyes will remain synchronized (conjugate gaze) when the head is turned from side to side. The eyes turn

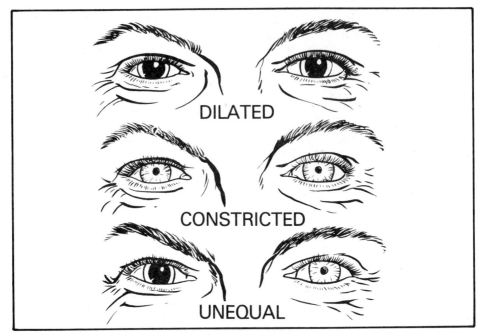

DILATED

CONSTRICTED

UNEQUAL

Figure 6-10. Pupils of the eyes.

in the opposite direction from the way the head is turned. Since this resembles the way a toy doll's eyes move, this test is called the *doll's eyes reflex*. (The proper name for the test is the oculocephalic reflex.) If this reflex is present, you can almost be certain that the brainstem is uninjured. This test is *never* done in the field on a trauma victim who may have a neck injury since turning the head from side to side would probably cause spinal injury with permanent paralysis.

Extremities

Note sensation and motor function in the extremities. Can the patient feel you touch his hands and feet? Can he wiggle his fingers and toes? If the victim is unconscious, note his response to pain. If he withdraws or localizes to the pinching of his fingers and toes, he has intact sensation and motor function. This is a sign of normal or only minimally impaired cortical function.

Both [decorticate posturing (arms flexed, legs extended)] and [decerebrate posturing (arms and legs extended)] are ominous signs of deep cerebral hemispheric or upper brainstem injury. Flaccid paralysis usually means spinal cord injury.

Decisions on management of the head trauma patient are made on the basis of changes in all of these different signs. You are establishing the baseline from which later judgments must be made: *record your observations.*

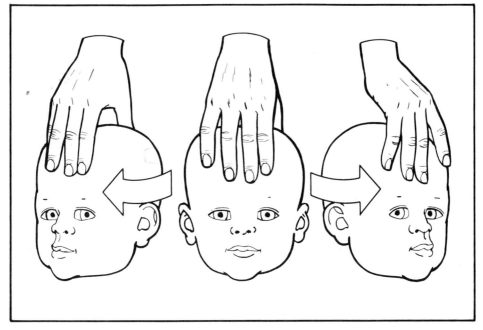

Figure 6-11. Doll's eyes reflex.

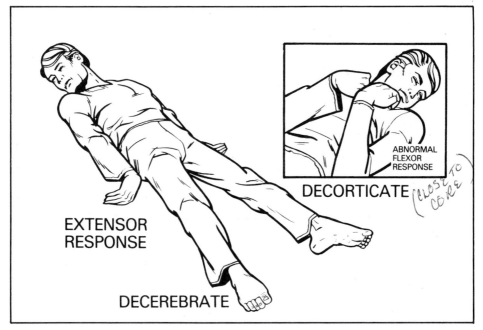

Figure 6-12. Decorticate and decerebrate posturing.

Management of the Head Trauma Victim

There is not a great deal that you can do for the head trauma patient in the field. It is most important to make a rapid assessment and then transport the victim to a facility capable of treating head trauma. The important points of management in the field are these:

1. Secure the airway and provide good oxygenation. The brain does not tolerate hypoxia, so good ventilation is mandatory. *The head injury patient should be hyperventilated.* This decreases intra-cranial pressure. The neck should be immobilized in a Philadel-phia collar or other good immobilization device (not a soft foam rubber choke collar). If the patient is comatose, he should be intubated. This prevents aspiration and provides better oxygen-ation.
2. Record baseline observations: This includes recording the level of consciousness, vital signs, pupils, and extremity movement and sensation. If the patient develops signs of shock, look for another cause.
3. Frequently monitor and record the observations listed above.
4. You may be ordered to start an intravenous line. Unless the pa-tient is in shock, the only purpose of an intravenous line should be to give medication. Fluids are restricted in head trauma.

Potential Problems

1. Convulsions: Head trauma, especially intracranial hemorrhage, may cause convulsions. The convulsing patient becomes hypoxic, so persistent seizure activity may worsen his condition. You may be ordered to give valium IV to stop the seizures.
2. Vomiting: A patient with head trauma almost always vomits. You must remain alert to this to prevent aspiration. If the patient is unconscious, he should be intubated. Otherwise, have suction available and be ready to log roll him on his side (maintaining immobilization of the cervical spine).
3. Rapidly deteriorating condition: A patient who shows rapid de-terioration of signs should be transported rapidly to improve chances for survival. There is nothing definitive you can do in the field. Call ahead so that a neurosurgeon can be available and the operating room prepared by the time you arrive at the hos-pital. Developing rapid field response will not make up for time lost getting the appropriate doctor to the hospital.
4. Shock: Think "spinal cord injury or bleeding."

Summary of Management

1. Stabilize the neck

2. Secure and maintain the airway
3. Hyperventilate
4. Record baseline vital signs, observations of pupils, and neurological examination
5. Continuously monitor and record
6. Transport

Glasgow Coma Scale

This is a simple way to evaluate and monitor the patient who is in coma from *head trauma*. It has good value in predicting the outcome. There are three components. Score by the best response.

Eye Opening
Spontaneous 4
To voice 3
To pain 2
None 1

Verbal Response
Oriented...................... 5
Confused 4
Curses........................ 3
Incomprehensible
    sounds 2
None 1

Motor Response
Obeys 6
Localizes..................... 5
Withdraws.................... 4
Flexion
    (decorticate).............. 3
Extension
    (decerebrate).............. 2
None 1

Total Scores
8 or better . . .
    94% favorable outcome
5, 6, 7 . . .
    50% favorable outcome
    (children 90%)
3 and 4 . . .
    10% favorable outcome
5, 6, 7 who drop a grade . . .
    100% unfavorable
    outcome
5, 6, 7 who improve to
    greater than 7 . . .
    80% favorable outcome

Chapter 7

Extremity Trauma

Fractures, dislocations, and soft tissue injuries of the extremities are often the most dramatic injuries apparent when first examining a victim, but such injuries, although often disabling, are rarely immediately life threatening. You must keep in mind the importance of treating life-threatening injuries first. Thus, airway, breathing, circulation, bleeding, and treatment of shock precede splinting of fractures.

Hemorrhagic shock is a potential danger of very few musculoskeletal injuries. Only direct lacerations of arteries or fractures of the pelvis or femur are commonly associated with sufficient bleeding to cause shock. Injuries to peripheral nerves or vessels causing neurovascular compromise are the most common complications of fractures and dislocations. Thus, evaluation of sensation and circulation (pulses, color) distal to fractures is very important.

I. **Injuries**
   A. Fractures: Fractures may be open (compound) with the broken end of the bone still protruding or having once protruded through the skin, or they may be closed (simple) with no communication to the outside. Open fractures have associated soft tissue injuries both from the initial trauma and from the cutting of tissue by sharp edges of broken bone. Significant amounts of blood can be lost into this injured soft tissue. A fracture of the lower leg can cause the loss of 1 to 1.5 units of blood into the surrounding tissue, a fractured femur can cause the loss of 2 units, and a fractured pelvis can cause the loss of 1 unit for each fracture (up to 20 units). Pelvic fractures that lacerate the large pelvic vessels can cause exsanguinating hemorrhage. Remember, multiple fractures can cause life-threatening hemorrhage without any *external* blood loss. Open fractures add the dangers of external hemorrhage and contamination of the wound with bacteria.
   B. Dislocations: Joint dislocations are extremely painful injuries. Major joint dislocations, though not life threatening, are often true emergencies because of neurovascular compromise that can, if not treated quickly, lead to amputation. It is very important to check for sensation, pallor, and pulses distal to

89

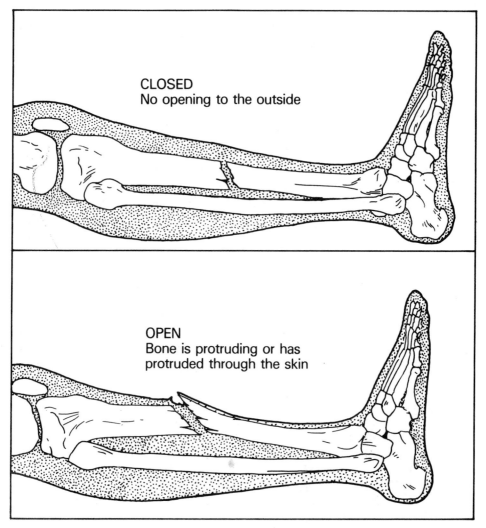

CLOSED
No opening to the outside

OPEN
Bone is protruding or has
protruded through the skin

Figure 7-1. Classification of fractures.

major joint dislocations. The normal rule is to splint joint injuries in the position that you find them. Pad and splint the extremity in the most comfortable position and rapidly transport the patient to a facility that has orthopedic care available.

C. Amputations: These are disabling and sometimes life-threatening injuries. The stump should be covered with sterile dressings and an elastic wrap. If bleeding cannot be controlled with pressure, a tourniquet may be used. If you can find the amputated part, bring it with you, but do not give the patient false hopes about reimplantation. Reimplantation is usually not done in patients with other major injuries, in patients over

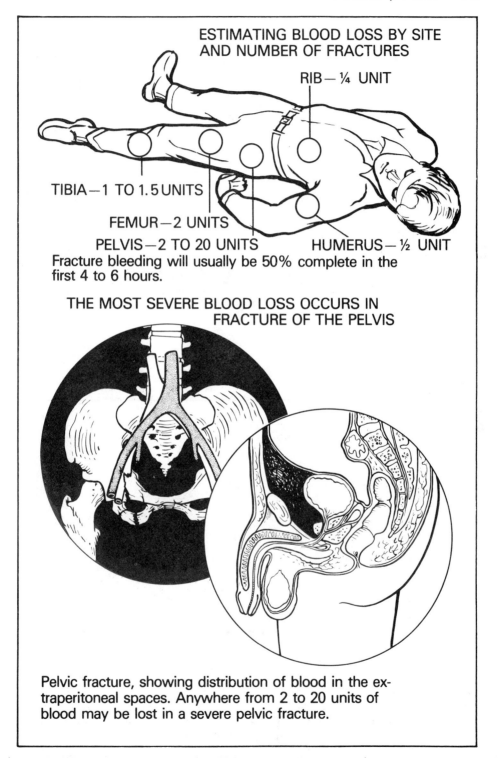

ESTIMATING BLOOD LOSS BY SITE
AND NUMBER OF FRACTURES

RIB — ¼ UNIT

TIBIA — 1 TO 1.5 UNITS

FEMUR — 2 UNITS

PELVIS — 2 TO 20 UNITS

HUMERUS — ½ UNIT

Fracture bleeding will usually be 50% complete in the
first 4 to 6 hours.

THE MOST SEVERE BLOOD LOSS OCCURS IN
FRACTURE OF THE PELVIS

Pelvic fracture, showing distribution of blood in the ex-
traperitoneal spaces. Anywhere from 2 to 20 units of
blood may be lost in a severe pelvic fracture.

Figure 7-2. Internal blood loss from fractures.

40 years of age, in avulsion or crush injuries, or in injuries to the lower extremities. Small amputated parts should be wrapped in a sterile dressing soaked in saline. If ice is available, seal the part in a small plastic bag and place it in a larger bag or container containing ice and water. Do not use ice alone and *never* use dry ice. Cooling the part will increase the viability from 4 to 6 hours to about 18 hours. It is important to bring amputated parts even if reimplantation is not feasible—some of the part may be used in the repair.

D.   Wounds: Cover wounds with a sterile dressing and bandage. Bleeding can be stopped with pressure dressings or pneumatic splints. Tourniquets are almost never needed.

E.   Neurovascular injuries: The nerves and major vessels generally run together and thus may be injured together. Loss of circulation and/or sensation can be due to swelling, disruption by missiles or broken bone ends, or compression by the bone fragments. Extremity pulses and sensation are always checked

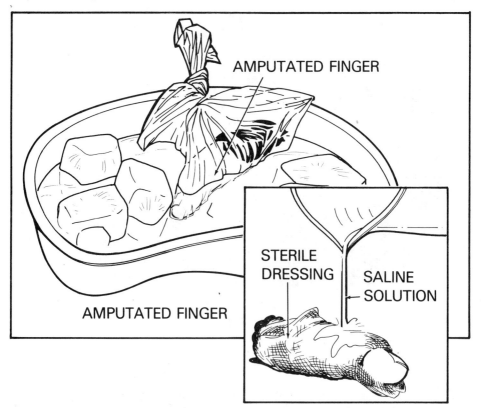

Figure 7-3. Transportation of amputated part. If ice and time are available, seal part in small container and place this in larger container of ice and water. Do *not* use dry ice. Do *not* place amputated part directly on ice. If no ice or time is available, wrap part in sterile dressing soaked in saline.

before and after straightening of fractures or after application of splints or traction.

F. Sprains and strains: These injuries cannot be differentiated from fractures in the field. Treat them as if they are fractures.

G. Impaled objects: Do not remove them. Apply padding and transport the patient with the object in place. The cheek of the face is the only exception to this rule.

II. **Assessment and Management**

A. History: This is especially important in extremity trauma. It is important to note the apparent mechanisms of injury and the position and condition of the extremity when you first arrive.

B. Assessment (general): During the secondary assessment, you should quickly palpate each extremity, looking for deformity and areas of spasm or tenderness. Check the joints for pain

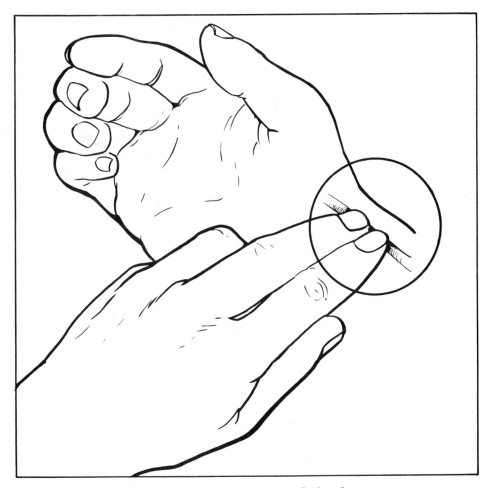

Figure 7-4a. Palpation of radial pulse.

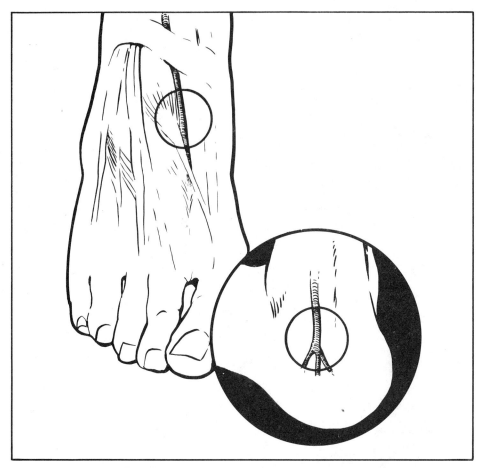

Figure 7-4b. Location of posterior tibial and dorsalis pedis pulses.

or movement. Check and record distal pulses and sensation. Crepitation or grating of bone ends is a definite sign of fracture, but you should not attempt to demonstrate it since you would be causing further injury to the soft tissue.

C. Management (general): Proper management of fractures and dislocations will decrease the incidence of serious complications and may well prevent the loss of an extremity. Treatment in the field is directed at proper immobilization of the injured part by use of a splint.

1. Purpose of splinting: The objective is to prevent motion in the broken bone ends, thereby preventing further damage to muscles, nerves, and blood vessels.

2. General rules of splinting:

    a. You must adequately visualize the injured part. Clothes should be cut off, not pulled off, unless there

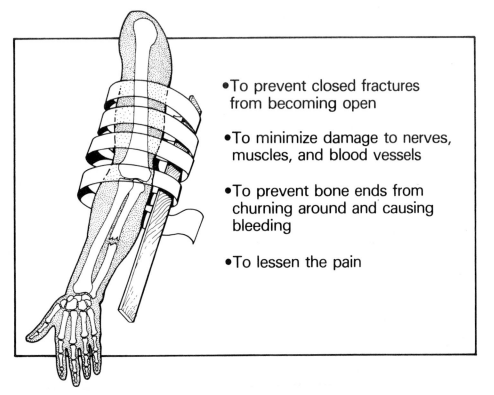

•To prevent closed fractures from becoming open

•To minimize damage to nerves, muscles, and blood vessels

•To prevent bone ends from churning around and causing bleeding

•To lessen the pain

Figure 7-5. Reasons for splinting.

is only an isolated injury that presents no problem with maintaining immobilization.

b. Check and record distal sensation and circulation before and after splinting. Check movement distal to the fracture if possible (e.g., ask the patient to wiggle his fingers).

c. If the extremity is severely angulated, you should apply gentle traction in an attempt to straighten it. If resistance is encountered, splint it in the angulated position.

d. Open wounds should be covered with a sterile dressing before you apply the splint.

e. Use a splint that will immobilize one joint above and below the injury.

f. Pad the splint well.

g. Do not attempt to push bone ends back under the skin. When you apply traction, if the bone end retracts back into the wound, allow it to do so but be sure to notify the receiving physician.

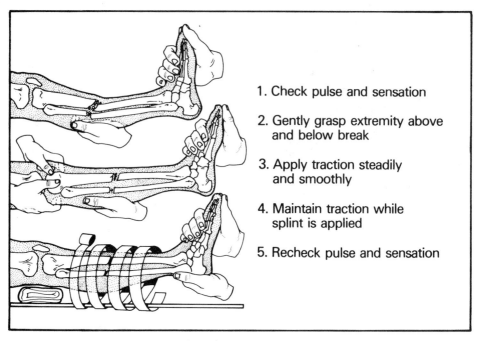

1. Check pulse and sensation

2. Gently grasp extremity above and below break

3. Apply traction steadily and smoothly

4. Maintain traction while splint is applied

5. Recheck pulse and sensation

Figure 7-6. Straightening angulated fractures.

    h.   Splint all injuries before moving the patient unless a life-threatening situation prevents it.

    i.   If in doubt, splint.

3. Types of splints:

    a.   Rigid splint: This type of splint can be made from many different materials such as cardboard, plastic, metal, or wood. It should be padded well and should always extend one joint above and below the fracture.

    b.   Soft splint: This type includes air splints, pillows, and slings and swathes.

        1) Air splints are good for fractures of the lower arm and lower leg. They have the advantage of compression to stop bleeding and swelling in the area they cover. You must blow these up by mouth (never a pump) until they give good support and yet can be easily dented with slight pressure from a fingertip. Remember that if they are applied in a cold environment, the pressure will increase as they warm up. The pressure also increases if they are applied on the ground and then the patient is transported by air. When you use air splints, you must constantly check the pressure to be sure that the splint is not getting too tight (or too loose—they often leak). There

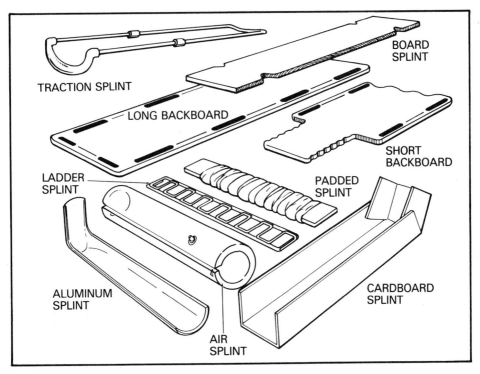

Figure 7-7a. Types of splints.

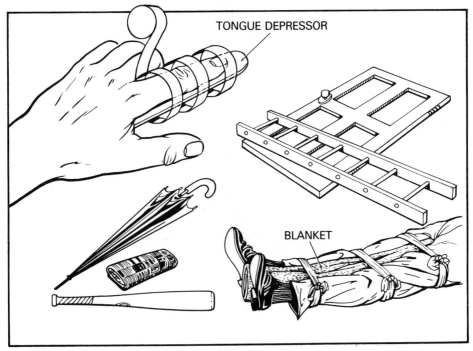

Figure 7-7b. Improvised splinting materials.

are two major disadvantages of air splints: you cannot monitor extremity pulses while they are on; the splints often stick to the skin and are painful to remove (they should be powdered).

2) Pillows make good splints for injuries to the ankle or foot. They are also helpful along with a sling and swathe to stabilize a dislocated shoulder.

3) Slings and swathes are excellent for injuries to the clavicle, shoulder, upper arm, elbow, and sometimes the forearm.

c. Traction splint: This device is designed for fractures of the lower extremities. It holds a fracture immobile by the application of a steady pull on the extremity. The most common are the Thomas, Sager, Hare, and Klippel splints. They are used to immobilize fractures of the femur and proximal tibia and fibula, and they work by applying counter traction to the ischium and groin. They must be padded and applied with care to prevent excessive pressure on the genitalia. You must also use care in applying the hitching device to the foot and ankle so as not to interfere with circulation.

D. Management (specific injuries)

1. Spine: This is covered elsewhere in the book but included here to remind you that if there is any chance of spinal

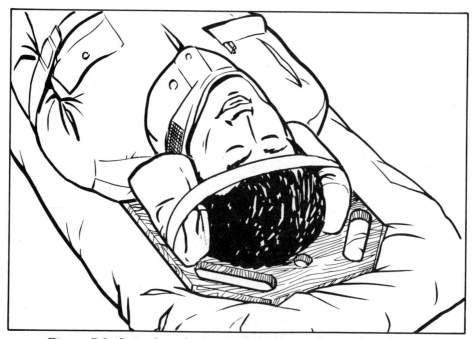

Figure 7-8. Spine board with Philadelphia collar and sandbags.

injury, proper immobilization must be done to prevent lifelong paralysis or even death from a spinal cord injury. Remember, a fall in which a victim lands on his feet may cause lumbar spine fracture.

2. Pelvis: While the pelvis is not an extremity, it is practical to include injuries to it here. These injuries are usually caused by motor vehicle accidents or by falls from a height. There is always the potential for serious hemorrhage in pelvic fractures, so shock should be expected and prepared for. There is a high (10%) incidence of injuries to the bladder or urethra associated with pelvic fractures, but there is little you can do for these injuries in the field. A patient with a pelvic injury should be transported on a spine board. Pelvic fractures can be associated with severe bleeding; therefore, anti-shock trousers should be used to splint and to tamponade bleeding.

3. Femur: The femur is the longest and heaviest bone in the body. It usually fractures at midshaft and often is an open fracture. There is usually significant bleeding by the heavy muscles of the thigh. Bilateral femur fractures can be associated with loss of 50% of the circulating blood volume, so be prepared for development of shock. Use a traction splint.

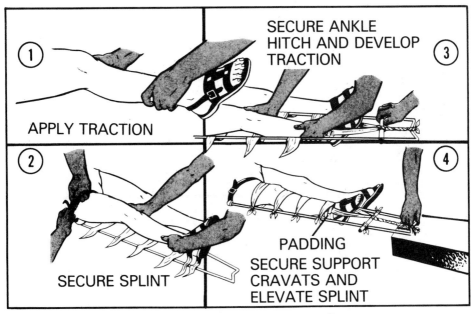

Figure 7-9a. Applying a traction splint.

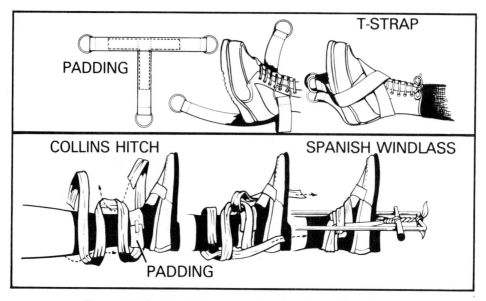

Figure 7-9b. Applying a traction hitch to the ankle.

4. Hip:
   a. Hip fractures are usually in the neck of the femur. These are probably the most common fractures in elderly people. The neck of the femur is very short and is completely surrounded by strong ligaments; thus, there is not much movement of the bone ends and little bleeding occurs. Because of the strength of the ligamentous structures, the fractured hip may still bear weight, but do not be fooled into thinking a fracture does not exist because the patient has walked with help. A traction splint is not necessary. The uninjured leg can be used to splint the fractured one. Hip fractures often refer pain to the knee, so always think of hip fracture when an elderly person falls and complains of knee pain only.
   b. Hip dislocation is a different story. Most hip dislocations are the results of car accidents in which the knee strikes the dashboard, forcing the hip out the posterior side of the joint. This is an orthopedic emergency and requires reduction as soon as possible to prevent sciatic nerve injury or necrosis of the femoral head. The hip will usually be flexed, and the victim will not be able to tolerate having the leg straightened. A hip dislocation should be supported in the most comfortable position by use of pillows and the

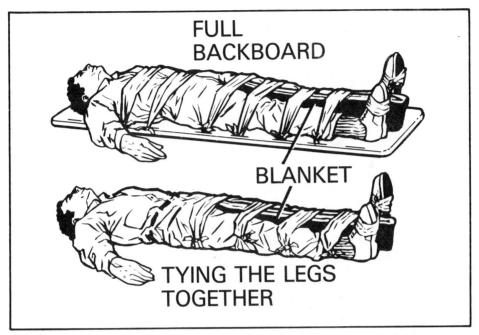

Figure 7-10. Hip fracture.

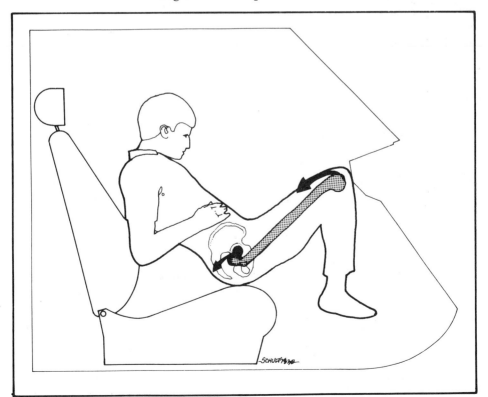

Figure 7-11. Mechanism of posterior dislocation of the hip.

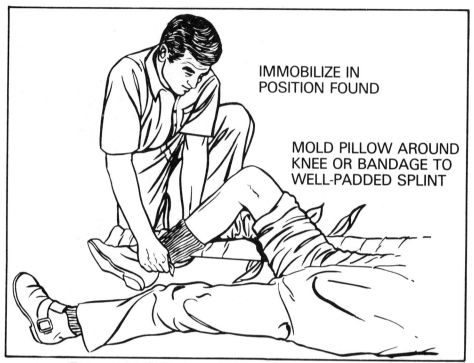

IMMOBILIZE IN
POSITION FOUND

MOLD PILLOW AROUND
KNEE OR BANDAGE TO
WELL-PADDED SPLINT

Figure 7-12. Splinting posterior dislocation of the hip.

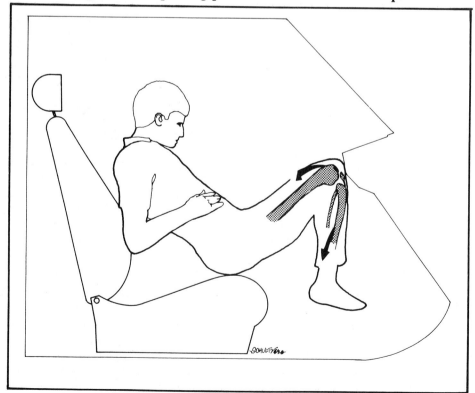

Figure 7-13. Mechanism of posterior dislocation of the knee.

uninjured leg. Transport the patient rapidly to a facility where orthopedic care is available.

5. Knee: Fractures or dislocations here are serious because the arteries are bound down above and below the knee and are often disrupted if the joint dislocates. About 50% of knee dislocations have associated vascular injuries, and many require amputation. Prompt reduction of knee dislocation is mandatory. You should apply gentle traction with a traction splint; many will easily reduce. If there is resistance to straightening the knee, splint it in the most comfortable position and transport the patient rapidly to a facility where orthopedic care is available. This is another true orthopedic emergency.

6. Tibia/fibula: Fractures of the lower leg are frequently the results of motorcycle or automobile accidents. They are often open and often have significant internal and/or external blood loss. Fractures of the upper tibia should be immobilized with a traction splint. Fractures of the lower tibia/fibula may be splinted with a rigid splint, air splint, or even a pillow.

7. Clavicle: This is the bone through which the upper extremity (arm) attaches to the central skeleton. It is the site of one of the most frequent fractures but rarely causes problems even though the subclavian artery and vein lie just beneath it. It is best immobilized in the field with a sling and swathe.

8. Shoulder: Most shoulder injuries are either a dislocation of the joint, a separation of the acromioclavicular joint,

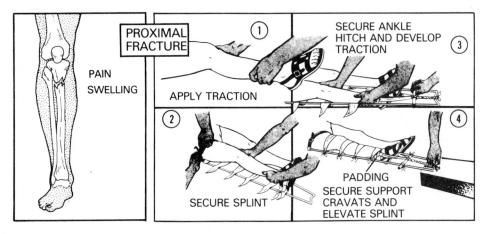

**Figure 7-14a. Splinting lower leg fractures.
Proximal fracture—traction splint.**

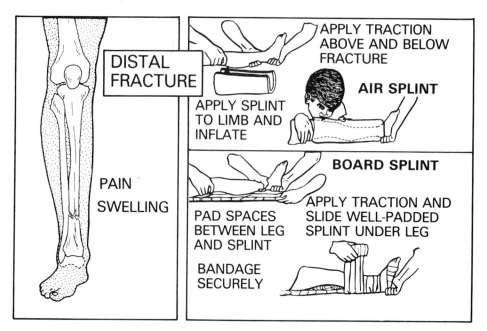

Figure 7-14b. Splinting lower leg fractures.
Distal fracture—air splint or board splint.

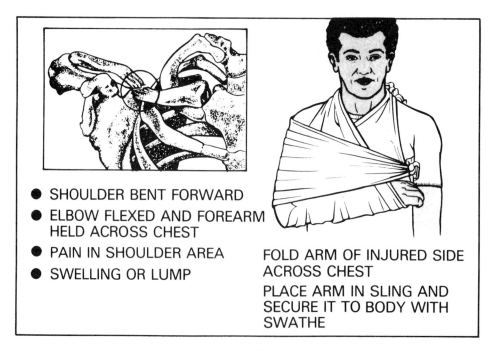

Figure 7-15. Fractured clavicle.

or a fracture of the upper humerus. A sling and swathe usually provides the best immobilization. Dislocated shoulders are very painful and often require a pillow between the arm and body to hold the upper arm at the most comfortable position.

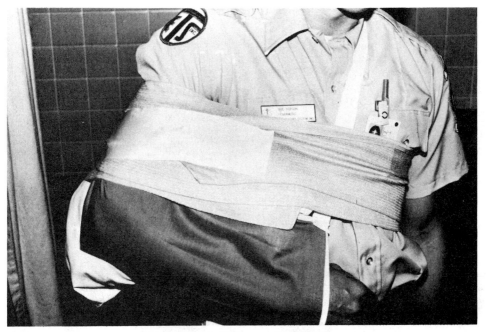

Figure 7-16. Dislocated shoulder.

9. Elbow: It is often difficult to tell whether there is a fracture or dislocation; both can be serious because of the danger of neurovascular injury. Elbow injuries should always be splinted in the most comfortable position and the patient rapidly transported for treatment. Do not attempt to straighten or apply traction to an elbow injury.

10. Forearm and wrist: This is a very common fracture, usually as a result of a fall on the outstretched arm. Usually, it is best immobilized with a rigid splint or an air splint. If a rigid splint is used, put a roll of gauze in the hand to hold it in the position of function.

11. Hand or foot: Industrial accidents involving the hand or foot often produce multiple open fractures and even avulsions. These injuries are often disabling and gruesome appearing but are usually not associated with life-threatening hemorrhage. A pillow is usually support enough for these injuries.

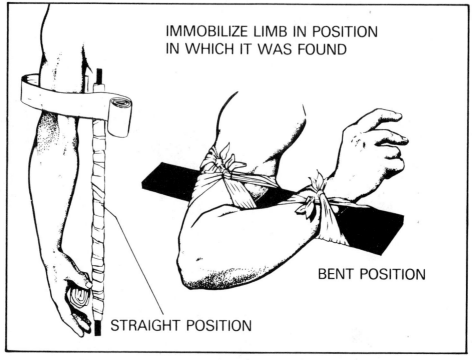

Figure 7-17. Fractures or dislocations of the elbow.

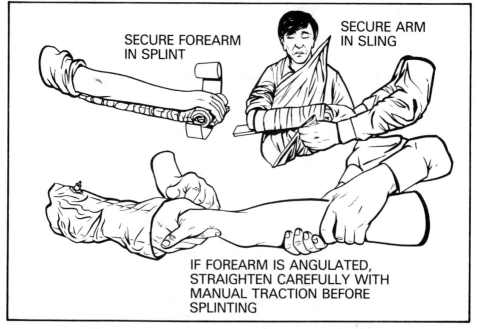

Figure 7-18. Fractures of the forearm and wrist.

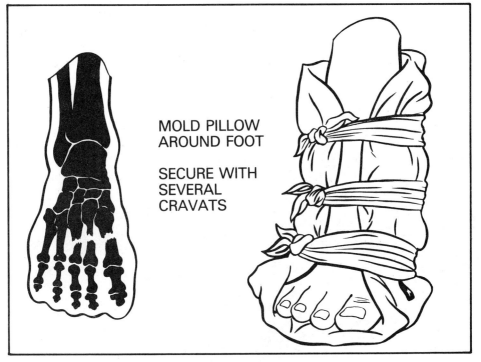

Figure 7-19. Fracture of the ankle or foot.

III. **Review of Important Points**
  A. Be alert to mechanisms of injury so that you know what fractures to suspect.
  B. Visualize the injured part.
  C. Be prepared for hemorrhagic shock in those fractures associated with significant bleeding.
  D. Always record sensation and circulation initially and after any manipulation or splinting.
  E. Pad splints well.
  F. Immobilize one joint above and below the fracture.
  G. Splint before moving.
  H. If in doubt, splint.
  I. Don't waste time. Be fast but be careful.

Chapter 8

Abdominal Trauma

Abdominal trauma may be blunt or penetrating. Most victims will live long enough to arrive at the hospital; most deaths occur because of a delay in diagnosis of intra-abdominal injury requiring surgery (surgery in first 12 hours: 12% mortality; surgery after 12 hours: 50% mortality). Only a small percentage of multiple trauma victims will have clinical signs and symptoms of abdominal injury (less than 3% in one study), but about 40% of these victims will have abdominal injuries severe enough to require surgery. Thus, it is important to have a high index of suspicion for abdominal injury and to record any changes noted during evaluation and transport. Those victims who have major abdominal vascular injuries bleed to death quickly. Studies have shown a marked increase in the survival rate of these victims when advanced life support techniques are begun in the field.

Anatomy

The abdomen contains the liver, spleen, pancreas, stomach, intestines, aorta, inferior vena cava, kidneys, bladder, lower vertebral column, pelvis, and spinal cord. In the woman there are also the ovaries and uterus. For practical purposes, the abdomen is divided into three areas for evaluation.

Intrathoracic Abdomen

This area is underneath the lower ribs and thus difficult to palpate. The liver, stomach, spleen, and diaphragm are found here. Injury to the lower ribs is often associated with injury to the underlying organs— especially the spleen.

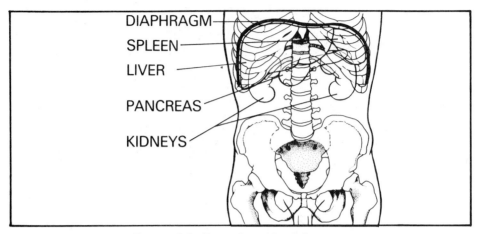

Figure 8-1. Intrathoracic abdomen.

True Abdomen

This is the area we commonly think of as the "abdomen." It contains the large and small intestines, the bladder, and, for practical purposes, the pelvis. Although this area is easier to examine, it is often difficult to decide between contusions of the abdominal wall and injury to the contents of the abdomen.

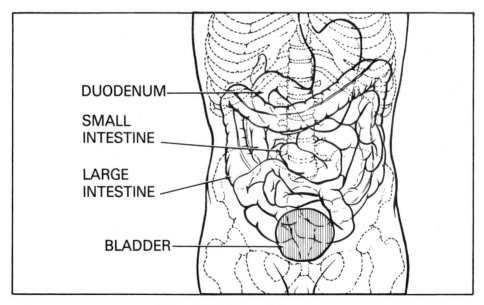

Figure 8-2. True abdomen.

Retroperitoneal Abdomen

This is the area behind the posterior peritoneum. It contains the pancreas and part of the duodenum, the abdominal aorta, inferior vena cava, kidneys, uterus, and, for practical purposes, the lower vertebral column and spinal cord. This area is very difficult to examine, and diagnosis of injuries often requires sophisticated procedures.

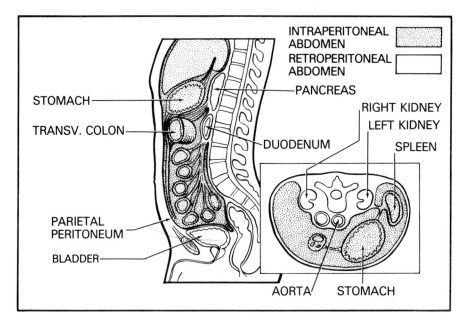

Figure 8-3. Retroperitoneal abdomen.

Types of Injuries

Penetrating Injuries

These can be from stab wounds or gunshot wounds. Injuries include the following:

1. Injuries to vessels, causing hemorrhage
2. Injuries to organs, causing hemorrhage
3. Injuries to organs, causing organ failure
4. Perforation of intestines
5. Protrusion of viscera through the wound

The first two types of injuries may present immediately as hypovolemic shock or may not show up for hours. The second two types of injuries will usually not present themselves for a period of time: usually hours or even days. Protrusion of viscera through the wound is, of course, immediately obvious. Thus, in penetrating injuries of the abdomen, your main, immediate concern is development of hypovolemic shock. Remember that a patient with a gunshot wound or stab wound (depending on the length of the instrument) of the chest, flank, or back may have an injury in the abdomen.

Blunt Abdominal Trauma

This injury can be from direct compression of the abdomen, with fracture of solid organs and blowout of hollow organs, or from deceleration, with tearing of organs or their blood vessels. As in penetrating injuries, the immediate danger to the patient is exsanguinating hemorrhage. A blunt abdominal injury frequently does not present with impressive signs and symptoms early, so you must keep a high index of suspicion to be prepared for the development of hemorrhagic shock.

Evaluation and Stabilization of the Patient with a Suspected Abdominal Injury

I. **Observation and History**
Develop the habit of critically appraising the scene of an accident to predict what type of injuries could have been sustained: poorly adjusted seat belts can cause rupture of the bladder or diaphragm, the steering wheel can cause abdominal as well as chest injuries, and broken window or door knobs can injure the abdomen or chest. Accidents in which the car has flipped over can result in injury to any system. If a stab wound occurred, how long was the instrument? If the patient was shot, was the trajectory of the bullet up or down? Your observation and questions at the scene can be extremely helpful later to the physician who must evaluate the patient at the emergency room.

II. **Examination**
First follow the ABCs. The abdomen is generally examined during the secondary examination. Use the standard (but modified) look, listen, and feel examination.
   A. Look: Look at the front, back, and sides of the abdomen. You may have to log roll the patient to get a good look. Notice if the abdomen is distended or if any bruises, abrasions, lacerations, puncture wounds, or protruding viscera are present.
   B. Do *not* listen: Listening for bowel sounds in the field is probably a waste of the golden hour. It can be done after the victim arrives at the hospital.
   C. Feel: Gently feel the anterior and posterior abdomen and record tenderness or masses. Do not worry about trying to

decide on specific injuries; that can be done at the emergency room. If there are any indications of abdominal injury, you must be prepared to treat hemorrhagic shock.

III. **Stabilization**

A. Protruding viscera should be covered with sterile dressings moistened with saline or water. Do not attempt to push the intestines back into the abdomen. You cannot use the abdominal section of MAST if viscera are protruding.

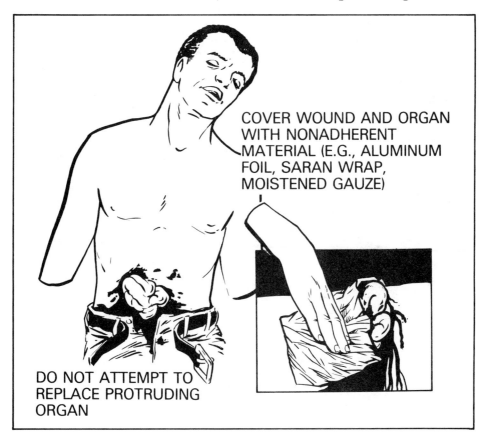

COVER WOUND AND ORGAN WITH NONADHERENT MATERIAL (E.G., ALUMINUM FOIL, SARAN WRAP, MOISTENED GAUZE)

DO NOT ATTEMPT TO REPLACE PROTRUDING ORGAN

Figure 8-4. Protruding intestines.

B. Any patient with a possible abdominal injury should have two large bore IVs started with Ringer's lactate and the MAST applied. The IVs may be at a keep-open rate initially and the MAST uninflated. The vital signs and clinical condition should be carefully watched; if signs of shock appear, fluid replacement should be begun immediately.

IV. **Important Points to Remember**

A. In the first hours after trauma, a tightly distended abdomen means massive intraperitoneal hemorrhage. This victim must have MAST and two IVs immediately, and you should call ahead to see that the surgeon and operating room are ready when you arrive.

B. A patient with hypotension, pallor, and tachycardia but no external injuries has bleeding into the abdomen or chest until proven otherwise.

C. Any gunshot or stab wound of the chest, flank, or back may have penetrated the abdomen.

D. Most deaths from abdominal trauma occur because of delayed diagnosis of a possible surgical abdomen. If your observation of the scene makes you think abdominal injury could have occurred, tell the receiving physician.

Chapter 9

Burns

A burn is an injury to tissue caused by direct thermal injury, exposure to a caustic chemical, or contact with an electrical current. Each year approximately 100,000 people require hospitalization from burns, and 12,000 die as the result of fires.

I. **Anatomy and Physiology**
   A. The skin is made up of two layers: the epidermis and the dermis. The epidermis or top layer of the skin mainly serves as a protective layer for the deeper structures. The dermis or deeper layer of the skin contains the hair follicles, sweat glands, oil glands, and sensory fibers for pain, touch, pressure, and temperature.
   B. Underneath the dermis is a layer of connective tissue and fat deposits called the subcutaneous tissue.

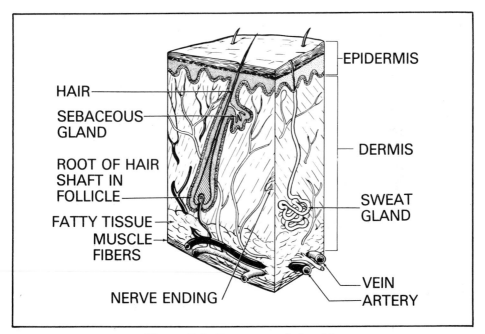

Figure 9-1. Structure of the skin.

C. The skin acts as an envelope to seal the body's fluids inside and germs outside. It is also an organ for sensation and temperature regulation and provides a flexible, mechanical, protective coat for the body.

II. **Pathophysiology**

A. When heat or caustic chemicals are applied to the skin, the layers are destroyed. The severity of the injury depends on the depth of the burn and the surface area involved as well as on associated injuries.

B. A first degree or superficial partial thickness burn involves only the epidermal layer. The skin is inflamed and tender and may peel in a few days, but it requires no treatment and heals without scarring.

C. A second degree or deep partial thickness burn involves the epidermis and part of the dermis but spares the deeper structures in the dermis from which new cells grow to form a new dermis and epidermis. These burns are painful, have either blisters or open weeping areas, and can lose a significant amount of fluid, but they usually heal within 14 to 21 days without scarring as long as infection does not develop.

D. A third degree or full thickness burn destroys the epidermis, dermis, and often even the subcutaneous layer or even deeper layers. These burns are white or charred and have a hard, leathery feel. All sensation is lost because the sensory organs

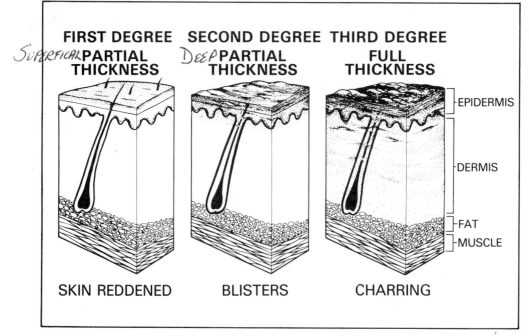

Figure 9-2. Classification of burns.

are destroyed. They are only painful around the edges where they taper into partial thickness burns. These burns heal by scar tissue formation and during healing fail to function as a protective barrier to fluid loss or bacteria.

E. Burn deaths usually occur due to smoke inhalation, hypovolemic shock, or overwhelming infection.

III. **Types of Burns**

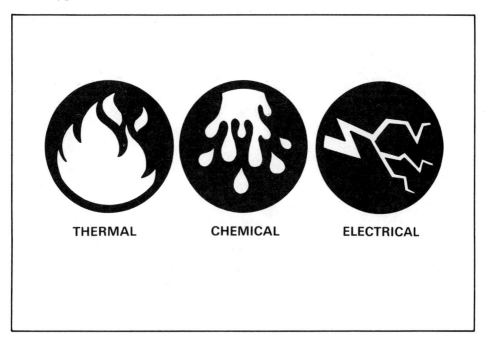

THERMAL   CHEMICAL   ELECTRICAL

Figure 9-3. Types of burns.

A. Thermal: Injury to the tissue is caused directly by heat. This may not only injure the skin but, if the victim inhales the flames, may cause injury to the upper airway. The upper airway filters, humidifies, and warms or cools the air we breathe. It performs this function so well that flames, even when breathed into the mouth and nose, almost never cause thermal injury beyond the pharynx and upper trachea. The injury to the upper airway causes swelling of the tissue and may cause complete airway obstruction. These symptoms may not present themselves for hours after the initial injury but may rapidly become life threatening when they do. All patients suspected of having thermal injury to the upper airway should be admitted to the hospital for close observation (about 30% of patients burned severely enough to require hospitalization have upper airway injury); there are certain situations and physical signs that should always alert you to this danger of upper airway injury:

1. Burns of the face
2. Singed eyebrows or nasal hairs
3. Burns in the mouth
4. Carbonaceous (sooty) sputum
5. History of unconsciousness
6. History of being confined in a closed space while being burned

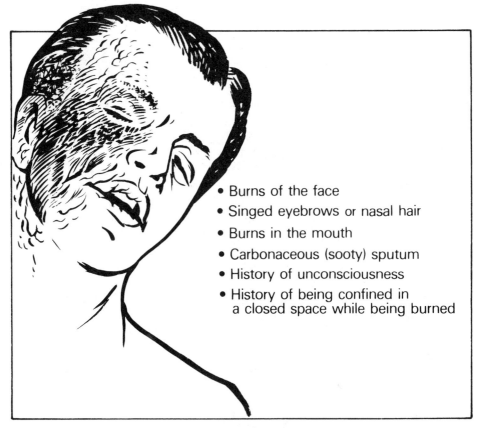

- Burns of the face
- Singed eyebrows or nasal hair
- Burns in the mouth
- Carbonaceous (sooty) sputum
- History of unconsciousness
- History of being confined in a closed space while being burned

Figure 9-4. Danger signs of upper airway injury.

B. Chemical: Chemical burns cause tissue injury from damage by strong acids, alkalis, or other corrosive materials. The severity depends on the type of corrosive, the concentration of the solution, the area involved, and the time it remains in contact with the skin. Alkalis are generally worse than acids because they penetrate the skin more quickly and are more difficult to remove.

C. Electrical: An electrical burn may cause direct damage from the electrical current or death from fibrillation of the heart.

It also causes sudden contraction of the muscles, so there may be musculoskeletal injuries as well. Usually, high voltage electrical burns have wounds of entrance and exit caused by the electric arc (temperature of 2,500 degrees centigrade) with varying amounts of injury inside the body between the two points. Electrical current inside the body tends to follow the blood vessels and nerves, causing vessel thrombosis and occlusion and tissue destruction. There may also be external thermal burns from the patient's clothing being ignited. It is impossible in the field to determine the amount of tissue damage because much of it may be inside the body. Thus, all patients with electrical burns should be transported to the hospital; most are admitted.

IV. **Associated Injuries**
  A. Smoke inhalation: There are approximately 12,000 burn deaths each year. At least one half of this number is due to smoke inhalation. There are over 200 toxic fumes produced

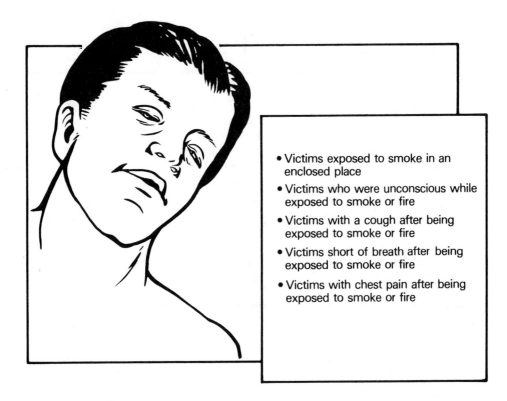

- Victims exposed to smoke in an enclosed place
- Victims who were unconscious while exposed to smoke or fire
- Victims with a cough after being exposed to smoke or fire
- Victims short of breath after being exposed to smoke or fire
- Victims with chest pain after being exposed to smoke or fire

Figure 9-5. Danger signs of inhalation injury.

from wood smoke and no one knows how many from synthetic products. The injury is usually to the alveoli where swelling occurs and edema fluid accumulates, preventing air exchange. The clinical picture is exactly like pulmonary edema of congestive heart failure. Most deaths occur at the scene from direct asphyxia, but many victims do not develop symptoms for up to 24 hours. All patients who were in a closed space, were unconscious, have a cough, or have shortness of breath or chest pain should be given oxygen and taken to the hospital for observation.

B.   Carbon monoxide poisoning: Fires in which there is not enough oxygen for complete combustion produce a gas called carbon monoxide. It is colorless, odorless, and tasteless, and if breathed into the lungs, it has an affinity for hemoglobin that is over 200 times greater than that of oxygen. Thus, carbon monoxide can saturate the hemoglobin molecules of the red blood cells so that they no longer can carry oxygen. The victim will thus die of hypoxemia. Generally, no symptoms develop until the blood is about 20% saturated at which time the victim complains of headache, nausea, and vomiting. At 30% saturation he becomes confused, and at 40% to 50% saturation coma occurs. Death occurs at higher concentrations. If the patient is simply removed from the source of the carbon monoxide, it will take about 5 hours for the carbon monoxide to clear from the blood. Administration of 100% oxygen decreases this to about 90 minutes, and a hyperbaric oxygen chamber can decrease the time to less than 30 minutes. The carbon monoxide–hemoglobin molecule is bright red, so a victim of this type of poisoning often has a "cherry-red" color. The most common sources of the gas are automobile engines, poorly vented heating devices, and fires in closed spaces.

C.   Explosion injury: Many fires are associated with explosions (e.g., propane gas explosions). Victims are often thrown some distance and may have fractures or internal injuries as well as burns. Chest injuries and inhalation injuries to the lungs are common in this type of accident.

V.   **Assessment of Burns**

A.   History: There are several things you should always record.

1.   What was the cause of the burn (an open flame, a chemical, a hot liquid)? It is very important to know the name and concentration of the chemical involved in chemical burns.

2.   Was an explosion involved? If so, you must expect and look for other injuries. Chest injuries are especially common here.

3. Was the victim in a closed space so that he may have inhaled smoke, steam, carbon monoxide, or flames?
4. Was the victim unconscious?
5. How long has it been since the burn occurred?
6. What has already been done for the burn? Was anything applied?
7. Past medical history: Does the victim have heart or lung disease or any other serious illness such as diabetes?
8. What medications is he taking?

B. Depth of burn: Estimate the depth from the appearance of the skin. Partial thickness burns are red or mottled, painful, and are blistered or swollen. Full thickness burns are leathery and may be translucent or white. The surface is usually dry and nontender. It is impossible to estimate the depth of chemical and electrical burns initially.

C. Extent of burn: In the field, estimation of burn size need only be a "ball park" figure. More precise determination of the size of the burn will be done at the hospital. What is important in the field is making the decision about which burned patients need to go to the hospital, and, if a burn center is in your area, which patients need to go directly there.

1. Rule of nines: A reasonable estimate of burn size can be made by dividing the body into areas of 9% or 18%. Notice that the head is proportionally larger in a child.

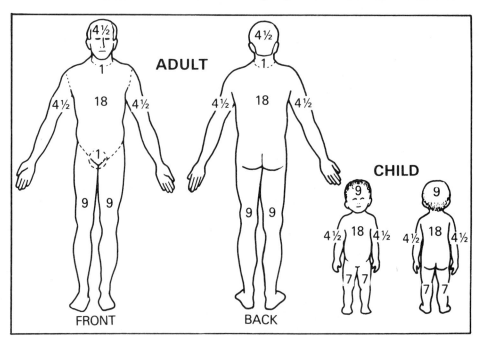

Figure 9-6. Rule of nines.

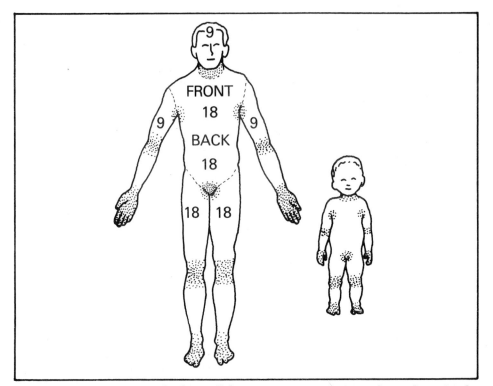

Figure 9-7. Areas in which small burns are more serious. Second or third degree burns in these areas (shaded portions) should be treated in the hospital.

For estimating the size of multiple or irregular burns, you can use the guide that the palm of the patient's hand is equal to about 1% of his body surface area.

2. Patients requiring hospital treatment:
   a. Any patient with a full thickness burn of more than 2% of body surface area
   b. Any patient with a partial thickness burn of more than 10% of body surface area
   c. Significant burns of face, hands, feet, or genitalia
   d. Burns that involve flexion areas such as neck, axilla, elbows, or knees
3. Patients that may need to be transported to a burn unit or burn center:
   a. Full thickness burns exceeding 10% of body surface area
   b. Partial thickness burns exceeding 20% of body surface area
   c. Serious burns of hands, feet, genitalia, or perianal area
   d. Inhalation injury

   e. Significant burns about the face

   f. High voltage electrical burns

   g. Burns associated with fractures or other major injury

   h. Lesser burns in patients who are already sick

  4. As a general rule, all burns should be seen by a doctor. Many partial thickness burns have become full thickness burns because of infection from lack of proper care.

VI. **Management of Burns**

 A. Thermal burns

  1. Remove the victim from the fire or the fire from the victim. This is one of the few exceptions to the normal ABCs of resuscitation. In many instances the speedy removal of the patient (and yourself) to a safe area must take priority over all else. Even in these cases remember that, if possible, the neck and back should be stabilized until you are sure no injury to the spine exists. Obviously, there will be times when this is not possible. You must consider your own safety during a rescue—dead EMTs don't save lives.

  2. Follow the ABCs of resuscitation.

  3. Stop the burning process. Cool the burn with tap water (use sterile water or normal saline if available) until the temperature is the same as normal skin. Do not apply ice water to extensive burns since this may cause hypothermia and worsen shock.

  4. Remove clothing and jewelry. Cut around clothing that sticks to the skin.

  5. Cover the burns with a clean sheet or sterile dressing. Do not apply any medications or ointments to the burn.

  6. Complete the secondary survey.

  7. Perform advanced life support as directed by Medical Control. Patients with burns involving more than 20% of body surface area will lose significant amounts of fluid through the injured area. This will not occur in the first few minutes after a burn, so unless prolonged transport is necessary, an IV is not absolutely indicated. If other injuries or shock dictates that an IV be started initially, Ringer's lactate is the fluid of choice. When starting an IV, do so in an area that is not burned. If burns cover all of the IV sites, you may start the IV in a burned area, but it will be very difficult to find a vein.

  8. If there is any chance of inhalation injury, give oxygen.

  9. Transport the patient.

 B. Chemical burns

  1. The most important field treatment is removing or diluting the chemical agent. Irrigation with a neutral

solution (water) must be carried out immediately. This should be done for 10 to 15 minutes at the scene. Use a water hose or shower: large volumes of water are needed. Do *not* try to neutralize acids with alkali or alkalis with acid; water is the only irrigant you should use. Clothes must be removed since they prevent removal of the chemical.

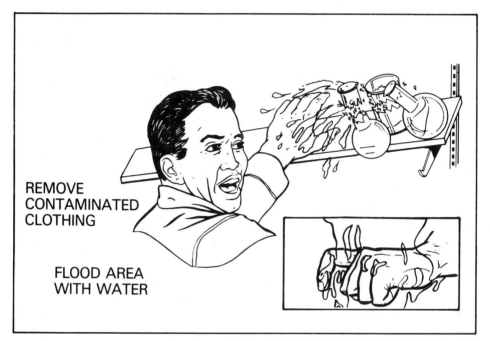

REMOVE CONTAMINATED CLOTHING

FLOOD AREA WITH WATER

Figure 9-8a. Chemical burns of the skin.

    2.   Dry lime or soda ash is a special case in that the addition of water causes a highly corrosive substance to form. The victim's clothes should be removed and the dry chemical brushed from his skin. If large volumes of water are available (hose or shower), the remainder of the chemical can be flushed away.

C.   Electrical burns: Here again is an exception to the routine ABCs of resuscitation.

    1.   The first priority in electrical burns is determining whether the patient is still in contact with the electrical source. If he is, you must remove him from contact without becoming a victim yourself. Handling high voltage electrical wires is **extremely** hazardous. Special training and special equipment are needed to deal with downed wires; you should *never* attempt to move wires with makeshift equipment. Tree limbs, pieces of wood, and

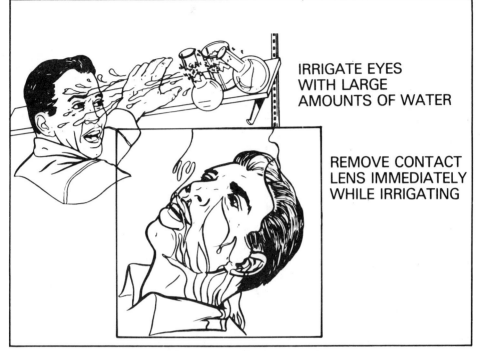

Figure 9-8b. Chemical burns of the eye.

IRRIGATE EYES
WITH LARGE
AMOUNTS OF WATER

REMOVE CONTACT
LENS IMMEDIATELY
WHILE IRRIGATING

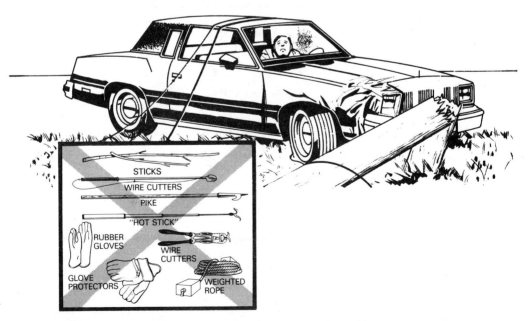

STICKS

WIRE CUTTERS

PIKE

"HOT STICK"

RUBBER
GLOVES

WIRE
CUTTERS

GLOVE
PROTECTORS

WEIGHTED
ROPE

Figure 9-9. Removal of high voltage electrical wires. *Do not* **try to remove wires with the safety equipment pictured (or with sticks) unless specially trained.** *Do* **turn off the electricity at the source or call the power company to remove the wires.**

even manila rope may conduct high voltage electricity. Even fire fighter's gloves and boots do not protect you in this situation. If possible, the handling of downed wires should be left to power company employees. An alternative is to develop a special training program with your local power company to learn how to use the special equipment needed to handle high voltage lines.

2. Cardiac arrest is a frequent complication of electrocution, so cardiopulmonary resuscitation is often necessary; use standard resuscitation procedures once the patient is free from the source of electricity.

3. All patients with electrical burns should have cardiac monitoring and an IV started in case antidysrhythmia drugs are needed.

4. All electrical burns are critical burns until proven otherwise.

VII. **Important Points to Remember**

A. Be alert at the scene: you must not become one of the victims.

B. Remember that burn victims often have other injuries as well.

C. Remember that inhalation injuries cause half of all burn deaths. The time to give oxygen is any time you think it might be needed.

D. Most burn victims, except victims of chemical burns, should rapidly be evaluated and transported. Chemical burns should be irrigated with water for 10 to 15 minutes unless other injuries dictate transport sooner.

Chapter 10

Trauma in Pregnancy

[Trauma, specifically that sustained in automobile accidents, is the leading cause of death among pregnant women.] Use of seat belts is *extremely* important for pregnant women, but the belts *must* be applied correctly. The lap belt must be worn low (below the uterus) and pulled tight across the pelvis (not abdomen). The shoulder belt is worn as usual. Proper use of belts helps prevent blunt injury to the uterus and fetus *and* protects the mother.

As professionals we must educate the public about the importance of seat belts in saving lives in automobile accidents. (We should also wear them ourselves since automobile accidents are also the leading cause of death among EMTs.)

I. **Changes During Pregnancy**
   A. During the first 3 months of pregnancy, the fetus is being formed. The fetus remains quite small, so there is little growth

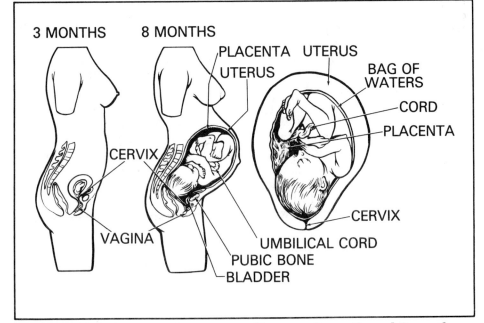

Figure 10-1. Anatomy of pregnancy. Uterus at 3 months and 8 months.

of the uterus during this period. After the third month, the uterus grows rapidly, reaching the umbilicus by the fifth month and the epigastrium by the seventh month.

B.   There are many other changes in the woman's body during this time. The blood volume is increased, the cardiac output increased, and the heart rate increased. The blood pressure is usually decreased slightly, and there is slowed peristalsis in the gastrointestinal tract. One very important change is the massive increase in the vascularity of the uterus and related structures.

II.   **Types of Injuries**

Obviously, the pregnant patient may sustain any injury that any other victim is subject to, but during the last two trimesters, the large uterus and fetus are particularly subject to certain injuries. Injuries to the uterus may be blunt or penetrating. In both cases the greatest danger to mother and baby is hemorrhage and hemorrhagic shock.

A.   Penetrating injuries: These are usually caused by gunshot or stab wounds. Since the uterus is anterior and usually quite large, it is frequently struck by penetrating objects. There are many very large blood vessels associated with the pregnant uterus, so massive hemorrhage may occur.

B.   Blunt trauma: The most common cause of this is automobile accident injuries, but falls or beatings also can cause injury. The uterus is well designed to protect the baby. The fetus is inside the body, inside a muscular chamber that is filled with fluid; these elements work together to provide a very efficient "shock absorber" so that most minor trauma to the abdomen, such as a blow or fall, does not harm the fetus. An automobile accident is a different story: the magnitude of force here is often great, and because of its size and location, the uterus is frequently injured. Sudden, blunt trauma to the abdomen during the later months of pregnancy may cause uterine rupture, abruptio placentae, premature labor, or severe bleeding from injury to the large vessels; other usual abdominal blunt trauma injuries, such as ruptured spleen or liver, may also occur. There is a good chance that rupture of the diaphragm will occur with blunt trauma during later pregnancy. Multiple trauma with fracture of the pelvis can cause laceration or tearing of the vessels in the pelvis with massive hemorrhage. The common problem with almost all of the blunt injuries to the pregnant abdomen or pelvis is massive bleeding and hemorrhagic shock.

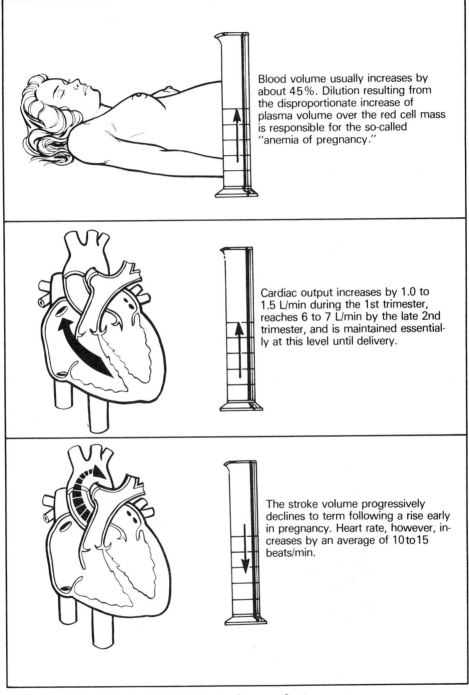

Blood volume usually increases by about 45%. Dilution resulting from the disproportionate increase of plasma volume over the red cell mass is responsible for the so-called "anemia of pregnancy."

Cardiac output increases by 1.0 to 1.5 L/min during the 1st trimester, reaches 6 to 7 L/min by the late 2nd trimester, and is maintained essentially at this level until delivery.

The stroke volume progressively declines to term following a rise early in pregnancy. Heart rate, however, increases by an average of 10 to 15 beats/min.

Figure 10-2. Physiologic changes during pregnancy.

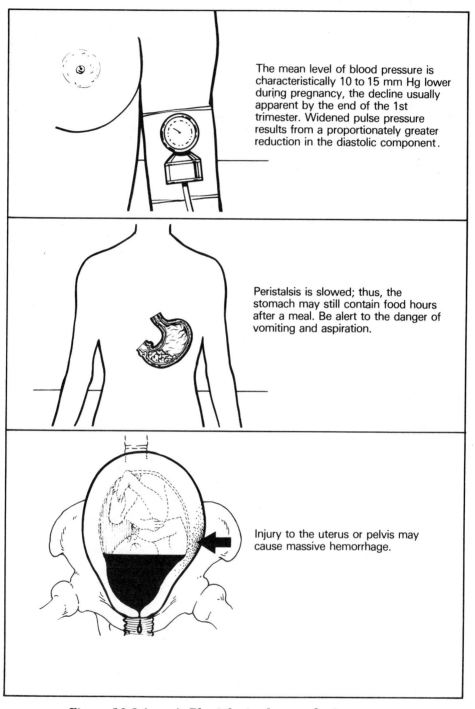

The mean level of blood pressure is characteristically 10 to 15 mm Hg lower during pregnancy, the decline usually apparent by the end of the 1st trimester. Widened pulse pressure results from a proportionately greater reduction in the diastolic component.

Peristalsis is slowed; thus, the stomach may still contain food hours after a meal. Be alert to the danger of vomiting and aspiration.

Injury to the uterus or pelvis may cause massive hemorrhage.

Figure 10-2 (cont.). Physiologic changes during pregnancy.

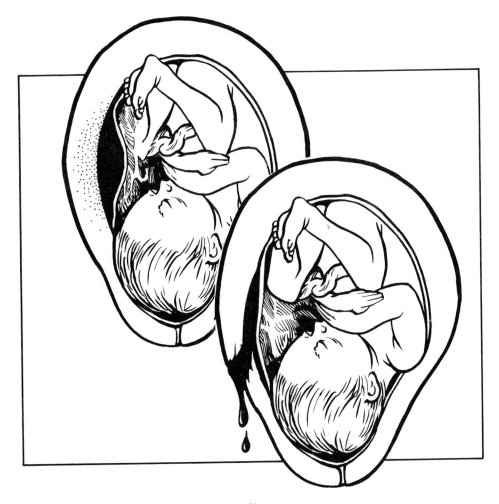

Figure 10-3. Blunt trauma to uterus. Blunt trauma may cause separation of the placenta or rupture of the uterus. Massive bleeding may occur.

III. Evaluation of the Pregnant Trauma Victim

A. The priorities are exactly the same.

Scene Survey →

1. Secure the airway and stabilize the spine
2. Assess breathing and circulation
3. Stop the bleeding
4. Treat the shock
5. Perform secondary survey, including neurological examination and splinting fractures
6. Transport with continuous monitoring

B. The things to remember are these:

1. The pregnant patient has a pulse that is 10 to 15 beats/min faster than normal, and the blood pressure is lower than normal (but with widened rather than narrowed

pulse pressure), so you may mistake the vital signs as being suggestive of shock when they are normal for the pregnant state.

2. The woman in later pregnancy may have a blood volume that is 20% to 45% higher than normal. This means she might lose much more blood internally before symptoms of shock appear. More volume is usually needed for fluid resuscitation of shock in pregnancy.

3. Because of the confusing vital signs in pregnancy and the extra blood volume, you *must be alert* or you will be late in diagnosing the development of hemorrhagic shock.

4. Trauma to the abdomen may cause occult intrauterine bleeding. Mark the top of the fundus with a marking pencil. Enlargement of the uterus suggests intrauterine bleeding.

5. Monitor vital signs frequently and watch the abdomen for signs of intra-abdominal bleeding.

IV. **Management of the Pregnant Trauma Victim**

Management of most injuries is the same as for those previously discussed, but there are certain things that are done differently.

A. Volume replacement: Hemorrhagic shock is the greatest danger from injuries to the uterus. The pregnant uterus is extremely vascular and can bleed profusely. If there is any doubt, ask for permission to start an IV of Ringer's lactate. Remember that increased volumes are often needed if shock occurs. MAST can be used, but inflate only the legs; inflation of the abdominal compartment cuts off blood flow to the baby.

B. Oxygen administration: The oxygen requirement of the woman in later pregnancy is 10% to 20% greater than normal, so if in doubt give oxygen.

C. Vomiting: Because of slow peristalsis and delayed gastric emptying, there is a greater chance of the patient vomiting and aspirating. Be ready.

D. Transport: If you transport a woman in later pregnancy on her back, the uterus will press on the inferior vena cava, obstructing the flow of blood back to the heart. This can be significant enough to cause hypotension, which is very dangerous to the baby. After the first 3 to 4 months of pregnancy, never transport the woman flat on her back. If there is no danger of spinal injury, you should transport her on her left side. If there is the danger of spinal injury, you may secure her to a long spine board, but prop the board up slightly on the right side so that the uterus is leaning to the left side; this prevents compression of the vena cava (which runs on the right side).

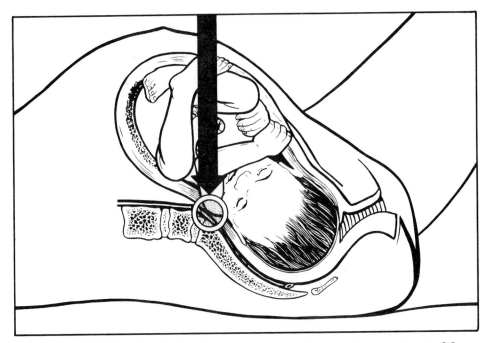

Figure 10-4. Venous return to the heart may be greatly compromised by uterine compression. Transport victim on her left side or tilt spine board to the left.

V. **Important Points to Remember**

A.   The most common cause of traumatic fetal death is death of the mother, so the goal of prehospital care is to get the mother to the emergency room alive, thus giving both the mother and the fetus the best chance for survival.

B.   Shock is more difficult to diagnose in the pregnant patient but is the most likely cause of prehospital death from injury to the uterus. It also requires more fluid to resuscitate because the mother has an increased blood volume.

C.   If there is any sign of hypoxia, give oxygen.

D.   Transport the patient on her left side or tilt the backboard so that she is leaning to the left; this prevents obstruction of the vena cava and makes aspiration less likely if she vomits.

Chapter 11

Pediatric Trauma

Trauma is the number one killer of children. After the neonatal period, 50% of childhood deaths are due to trauma.

As stated earlier, the general priorities are the same for children as for adults, but children are not simply "little adults." You must keep in mind the differences when evaluating and treating the injured infant or child.

To appreciate the abnormal you must learn the normal. Since children come in all sizes, you must remember some generalizations about various age groups.

Average Weights

Dosages of fluids and drugs are based on body weight. Since you do not have scales in the ambulance, you will usually have to estimate the weight of injured children. You should practice and develop your ability to do this.

Average Weights for Children

Age	Weight	
	lbs.	kg
Neonate (term)	7.5	3.5
6 months	15	7
1 year	22	10
2 years	30	13
3 years	33	15
4 years	37	17
5 years	40	18
6 years	48	22
8 years	60	27
10 years	73	33
12 years	84	38
14 years	110	50

Respiratory Rates

Respiratory rate is influenced by many factors such as fear, shock, drugs, or head injury. While important, it is not as useful as some of the other signs.

Normal Respiratory Rates

1. Infant: 40–60 per minute
2. Young child: 20–30 per minute
3. Older child: 12–20 per minute

Blood Pressure

The blood pressure is difficult to obtain in a small child. You must have a cuff that has a width of about three quarters of the width of the child's upper arm in order to obtain an accurate blood pressure. You may even need a doppler to hear accurate blood pressure. However, most ambulances are not equipped to obtain accurate blood pressure readings in small children. You must therefore learn to diagnose shock by observation of other signs.

Hypotensive Values

1. Neonate: less than 50 mm Hg
2. Infant: less than 60 mm Hg
3. Child (up to age 6): less than 70 mm Hg
4. Child (older than 6): less than 90 mm Hg

Heart Rate

While easily measured, this value is often influenced by fright (catecholamine release). Repeated determinations are important.

Tachycardia Values

Age	Upper Limit of Normal
Under 1 year	200
1–2 years	160
2–6 years	120
6–10 years	110
Older than 10	100

Airway and Ventilation

The small child has a large head and a short neck. His mandible is relatively small and his tongue relatively large. This makes mouth breathing difficult. Up to about the age of 6 months, infants can only breathe through their mouths when they are crying. Endotracheal intubation can be very difficult, especially in the traumatized child who must have his spine protected. If adequate ventilation can be accomplished without intubation, it is advisable to delay attempts at endotracheal intubation until the victim is in the more controlled environment of the hospital.

Diagnosis of Airway Obstruction

Observation is very important in diagnosing both the type and etiology of airway obstruction. You should note the rate and depth of respiration. Look for nasal flaring and intercostal as well as sternal and supraclavicular retractions. Listen for wheezing, grunting, snoring, or stridor. Notice whether the ribs are used in respiration or whether there is diaphragmatic breathing only. Notice skin color and sensorium; the hypoxic child will be cyanotic and either agitated (early hypoxia or fear) or lethargic (late hypoxia).

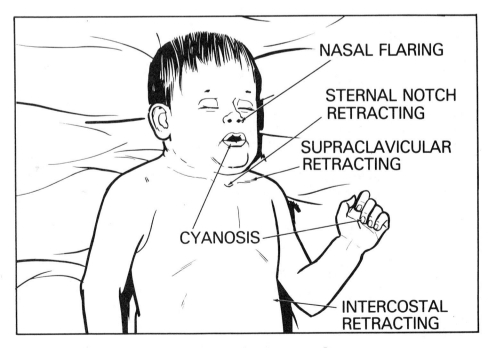

Figure 11-1. Signs of respiratory distress.

Normal respiration is not audible. When you hear abnormal breath sounds, you should think of airway obstruction.

[Wheezing is most commonly heard during expiration.] It may be from bronchospasm (asthma), but it may also be from airway obstruction due to other causes such as edema or foreign body aspiration.

[Grunting with expiration is heard most commonly in infants with partial airway obstruction.] It should be noted with alarm for complete airway obstruction can follow.

[Snoring is caused by oropharyngeal or nasopharyngeal partial obstruction.] It is most commonly caused by the tongue falling back into the posterior pharynx in the unconscious victim.

Stridor is usually harsh and high pitched. It is most commonly heard on inhalation.[Stridor is a sign of tight upper airway obstruction such as laryngeal edema.]

Injuries to the airways are not common during infancy and childhood, but those seen most often in the prehospital environment are the following:

1. Foreign body aspiration: Half of all cases are caused by peanuts. Children should not eat peanuts except those found in peanut butter.
2. Impact injuries to the face or neck: These may cause airway obstruction from edema or from actual laryngotracheal disruption. There can be compression of the airways and severe respiratory distress with only minimal external signs of soft tissue injury to the neck.
3. Chemical or thermal burns: The upper airways are so small in children that minimal swelling can cause major airway obstructions.

In general, mouth-to-mouth ventilation is best for children. You can stabilize the head and neck, open the airway with a jaw thrust, and give good ventilations without assistance from another rescuer. Using a bag-valve mask requires two rescuers to maintain head and neck stability as well as good face seal and ventilations. It is difficult to judge airway compliance using the bag-valve mask. You are more likely to hypoventilate since airway resistance may be many times higher in a child than in an adult. Bag-valve masks, if used, should not have a pop-off valve.

Keep suction available since vomiting and aspiration are much more common in children than in adults.

If you must do endotracheal intubation in a child, the external nares are your quickest guide to the size ET tube you should use. Remember that the tube must be secured well to prevent it from sliding down into the right mainstem bronchus or from pulling out of the larynx. The head must be stabilized in a neutral position to protect the spine and to prevent movement of the ET tube. In a small child, flexion or

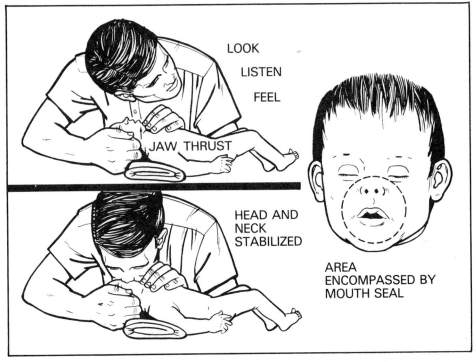

LOOK

LISTEN

FEEL

JAW THRUST

HEAD AND
NECK
STABILIZED

AREA
ENCOMPASSED BY
MOUTH SEAL

Figure 11-2. Mouth-to-mouth ventilation in a child.

extension of the head will cause sufficient movement of the ET tube to push it into the bronchus or pull it out of the larynx. Remember, cuffed ET tubes are not used in children younger than 7 years of age.

Chest Trauma

An important difference (from adults) is that children's ribs are so flexible that flail chest is uncommon. Pulmonary contusions and diaphragmatic hernias are more common because children are more commonly run over by wheels. Be very alert for development of tension pneumothorax. Needle decompression can be lifesaving. The technique is the same as that taught in the skill station.

Shock

Circulating blood volume is only 7% to 8% of body weight, so a small blood loss in a child may be sufficient to cause hemorrhagic shock. A 1-year-old child (10 kg) with a 2-inch laceration will bleed just as much as an adult (70 kg) with the same laceration. The adult has 5,000 cc of circulating blood volume whereas the child has only 750 cc. If each bled 200 cc from his wound, the adult would have no ill effects, but the child would be in obvious hemorrhagic shock.

The diagnosis of shock in a child requires careful observation. The most important signs are the following:

1. Pallor (secondary to decreased skin perfusion)
2. Altered sensorium (secondary to decreased brain perfusion)

Blood pressure is difficult to determine accurately in the small child so is of little use in the diagnosis of shock.

It is common for the traumatized child to bleed into shock from intrathoracic or intra-abdominal hemorrhage with no external blood loss.

Insertion of intravenous lines may be very difficult in the shocky child. In a small child the extremities can be wrapped with elastic bandages to achieve the same results as anti-shock trousers. A larger child may have pediatric MAST applied.

If you are able to start an intravenous line on the child in shock, you should give 10 cc/kg of Ringer's lactate over a few minutes. If the child does not improve, repeat 10 cc/kg.

In general, unless you have an extended transport time to the hospital, you should not spend time in the field attempting intravenous cannulation. You should load the victim and transport. Elastic wraps or MAST can be applied in the ambulance.

All children with shock should receive 100% oxygen if possible.

All children with shock should be wrapped to prevent hypothermia.

Spinal Cord Trauma

The same principles apply for children as for adults. Spinal cord injury is less common in children but does occur. Children should have their spines stabilized.

Head Trauma

Head trauma is the major cause of death from trauma in children. However, children with severe head injuries have a better chance of surviving with a good neurological recovery than do adults with the same types of injuries. Adults with decerebrate posturing have a grim prognosis, but over 80% of children with decerebrate posturing will survive. Most children with a Glasgow Coma Scale of 5 to 7 will live with a good functional recovery. Only 50% of adults will do well. The point here is that you must be aggressive in trying to save the child with what appears to be a severe head injury.

The most common pathological finding for children who die of brain injury is a diffuse swelling of the brain. This swelling seems to be from an increase in cerebral blood volume and not from edema fluid (edema is a later problem). In children the initial response of the injured brain is vasodilatation with increased cerebral blood flow and increased cerebral blood volume. This causes increased intracranial pressure, which causes pressure on brain structures. This, in turn, causes coma, respiratory arrest, and finally death.

Survival of children with head injuries depends on lowering intracranial pressure. Since this pressure is caused by increased cerebral blood flow, the treatment is to constrict the cerebral vessels. This decreases cerebral blood flow and decreases intracerebral pressure.

Hyperventilation is the best method for achieving cerebral vasoconstriction. You can begin hyperventilation in the field. Within minutes after lowering the $PaCO_2$ (from 40 torr to 25 torr), the intracerebral pressure will decrease. This early lowering of intracerebral pressure is a critical part of the therapy of head injuries. If children with possible head injuries begin to develop altered sensorium, you should begin hyperventilation with 100% oxygen immediately.

Remember that spinal cord injuries are more common in head injury victims. Usually, a victim with even a severe head injury will have some motion of his extremities. If the arms and legs are flaccid, you should expect spinal cord injury.

Extremity Trauma

The principles are the same as for adults. Small children usually do not require traction splints for leg fractures.

Abdominal Trauma

Blunt trauma is most common in small children. Liver injury is more common in children because the liver is relatively larger than in adults. Liver injuries are second only to head injuries as the major cause of death in children from trauma. Be very suspicious for abdominal injury in children. Any abdominal tenderness should alert you to be prepared for the development of hemorrhagic shock.

Burns

The principles are the same as for adults. Be aware especially of inhalation injuries since even slight swelling can cause airway obstruction in children.

General Approach to the Injured Child

The priorities are the same as for adults:

1. Airway maintenance and control of cervical spine
2. Assessment of breathing and circulation
3. Control of hemorrhage
4. Treatment of shock
5. Secondary survey and splinting of fractures
6. Transport with continuous monitoring

As a general rule, you should not separate the injured child from his parent(s) if possible. If the parent(s) and the child are both seriously injured, you may require two ambulances to properly care for each of them.

Children are so portable that they can (and should) be transported rapidly. There are *very few* procedures that should be done in the field. Often, a child may be packaged and sent by automobile before the ambulance arrives. One recent study found that most injured children, if transported by automobile, could have been in the emergency room before the ambulance arrived at the scene. We should therefore teach the lay public how to stabilize the child's spine during transport in an automobile.

Remember that children are often more frightened than adults. Talk gently to them and handle them gently.

Pediatric Drugs and Dosages

Weight	Sodium Bicarbonate (1 mEq/mL)		Epinephrine (1:10,000)		Atropine (0.1 mg/mL)	
	Dose	Volume	Dose	Volume	Dose	Volume
1 kg (2.2 lbs.)	1 mEq	1 mL	0.01 mg	0.1 mL	0.01 mg	0.1 mL
5 kg (11 lbs.)	5 mEq	5 mL	0.05 mg	0.5 mL	0.05 mg	0.5 mL
7.5 kg (16.5 lbs.)	7.5 mEq	7.5 mL	0.075 mg	0.75 mL	0.075 mg	0.75 mL
10 kg (22 lbs.)	10 mEq	10 mL	0.1 mg	1.0 mL	0.1 mg	1.0 mL
12.5 kg (27 lbs.)	12.5 mEq	12.5 mL	0.12 mg	1.25 mL	0.12 mg	1.25 mL
15 kg (33 lbs.)	15 mEq	15 mL	0.15 mg	1.5 mL	0.15 mg	1.5 mL
20 kg (44 lbs.)	20 mEq	20 mL	0.2 mg	2.0 mL	0.2 mg	2.0 mL
25 kg (55 lbs.)	25 mEq	25 mL	0.25 mg	2.5 mL	0.25 mg	2.5 mL
30 kg (66 lbs.)	30 mEq	30 mL	0.3 mg	3.0 mL	0.3 mg	3.0 mL
35 kg (77 lbs.)	35 mEq	35 mL	0.35 mg	3.5 mL	0.35 mg	3.5 mL
40 kg (88 lbs.)	40 mEq	40 mL	0.4 mg	4.0 mL	0.4 mg	4.0 mL
50 kg (110 lbs.)	50 mEq	50 mL	0.5 mg	5.0 mL	0.5 mg	5.0 mL

Pediatric Drugs and Dosages (cont.)

Weight	Lidocaine 1% (10 mg / mL)		Dextrose 50% (dilute 1:1 with sterile water for injection)		Naloxone (0.4 mg / mL)	
	Dose	Volume	Dose	Volume	Dose	Volume
1 kg (2.2 lbs.)	1.0 mg	0.1 mL	0.5 G	1.0 mL	0.01 mg	0.025 mL
5 kg (11 lbs.)	5.0 mg	0.5 mL	2.5 G	5.0 mL	0.05 mg	0.125 mL
7.5 kg (16.5 lbs.)	7.5 mg	0.75 mL	3.75 G	7.5 mL	0.075 mg	0.19 mL
10 kg (22 lbs.)	10.0 mg	1.0 mL	5.0 G	10.0 mL	0.1 mg	0.25 mL
12.5 kg (27 lbs.)	12.5 mg	1.25 mL	6.25 G	12.5 mL	0.12 mg	0.3 mL
15 kg (33 lbs.)	15.0 mg	1.5 mL	7.5 G	15.0 mL	0.15 mg	0.38 mL
20 kg (44 lbs.)	20.0 mg	2.0 mL	10.0 G	20.0 mL	0.2 mg	0.5 mL
25 kg (55 lbs.)	25.0 mg	2.5 mL	12.5 G	25.0 mL	0.25 mg	0.62 mL
30 kg (66 lbs.)	30.0 mg	3.0 mL	15.0 G	30.0 mL	0.3 mg	0.75 mL
35 kg (77 lbs.)	35.0 mg	3.5 mL	17.5 G	35.0 mL	0.35 mg	0.9 mL
40 kg (88 lbs.)	40.0 mg	4.0 mL	20.0 G	40.0 mL	0.4 mg	1.0 mL
50 kg (110 lbs.)	50.0 mg	5.0 mL	50.0 G	50.0 mL	0.4 mg	1.0 mL

Pediatric Defibrillation: 2 joules / kg

Chapter 12

The Trauma Cardiorespiratory Arrest

Advanced cardiopulmonary resuscitation has always been directed toward dealing with a cardiac cause of the cardiorespiratory arrest. In the trauma situation cardiac arrest is usually *not* due to myocardial infarction or coronary artery disease. The treatment must be directed at the underlying cause of the arrest or you will almost never be successful in your resuscitation efforts.

Causes of Cardiac Arrest Following Trauma

1. Hypoxia
   a. Airway obstruction
   b. Smoke inhalation
   c. Respiratory arrest secondary to head injury
   d. Respiratory arrest secondary to spinal injury
   e. Carbon monoxide poisoning
   f. Near drowning
2. Hemorrhagic shock (empty heart syndrome)
3. Tension pneumothorax
4. Pericardial tamponade
5. Electric shock
6. Myocardial contusion

Hypoxia

This is the most common cause of the trauma cardiorespiratory arrest. If you open the airway and ventilate with 100% oxygen, you may then follow standard advanced cardiac life support (ACLS) protocol in treating the arrest. Victims of head injury who have respiratory arrest usually do not survive; however, you should attempt resuscitation. Victims of spinal cord injury who have respiratory arrest (cervical spine fracture above C-3) will quickly respond to ventilation if they have not been

145

anoxic too long. Near-drowning victims should be ventilated with 100% oxygen. A significant number (19% in one study) of near-drowning victims who appear lifeless in the field will eventually have a complete recovery.

Hemorrhagic Shock (Empty Heart Syndrome)

This is another common cause of the trauma cardiorespiratory arrest. Like hypoxia, it is easily treatable. The treatment consists of oxygen, MAST, and intravenous fluids. The victim is invariably acidotic, so two ampules of $NaHCO_3$ should be given when the IVs are started. The most important drugs are 100% oxygen and replacement fluids, and then blood. Standard ACLS protocol may be used for dysrhythmias but will not take the place of fluid replacement. Aggressive treatment will save this victim.

Tension Pneumothorax

A frequently missed cause of cardiac arrest following trauma is the tension pneumothorax. Alert diagnosis and rapid needle decompression will usually be lifesaving. Give oxygen (100%) and have a chest surgeon standing by when you arrive at the emergency room.

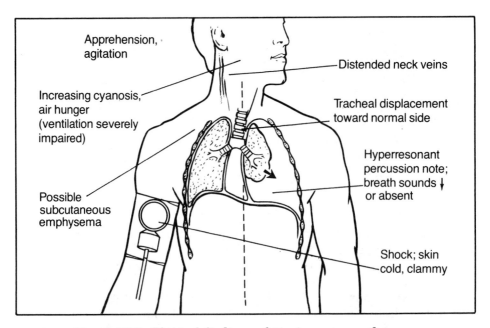

Figure 12-1. Physical findings of tension pneumothorax.

Pericardial Tamponade

The victim may appear to be in electromechanical dissociation (EMD) because the cardiac output is so low. The heart is squeezed by the blood in the pericardial sac until only a tiny amount of blood flows from the heart with each beat. The main clinical features are profound shock with distended neck veins and bilateral breath sounds. If the neck veins are not distended (some do not), the victim will appear to be in EMD but will not respond to ACLS measures. The only thing you can try to do in the field is to increase the filling pressure of the heart by using MAST and intravenous fluids. Rapid transport is absolutely essential if the victim is to survive. This condition is often difficult to diagnose in the field; suspect it when there are penetrating wounds of the chest or upper abdomen or if there are contusions of the anterior chest or sternum.

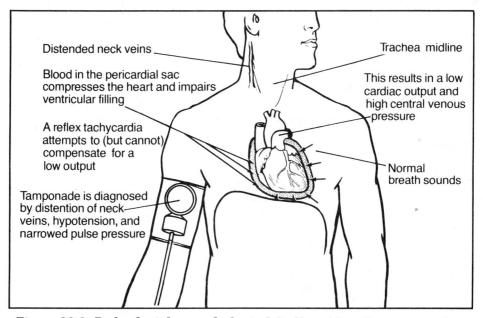

Figure 12-2. Pathophysiology and physical findings of cardiac tamponade.

Electric Shock

This usually presents as ventricular fibrillation. It responds readily to ACLS protocol if you arrive in time. Do not forget to stabilize the spine. Victims of high voltage electrical shock have often fallen from power poles or have been thrown several feet by the violent muscle spasm associated with the shock. Be sure the victim is no longer in contact with the electricity source. **Do not become a victim yourself!**

Myocardial Contusion

The victim has usually been in a deceleration accident. He may have a contusion of the chest or the sternum. This may present with any dysrhythmia depending on the size and area of damage to the heart. Use standard ACLS protocol. Remember, the victim may develop pericardial tamponade.

Approach to Trauma Victims in Cardiac Arrest

This is a special group of victims. Most are young and do not have preexisting cardiac conditions or disease. Because of this, they should have a good resuscitation rate. The extremely poor resuscitation rate for trauma victims in cardiac arrest is probably due to the fact that we approach these victims in the same way as we do those whose arrests are due to myocardial infarction.

Important Points in the Management of Victims of Trauma Cardiorespiratory Arrest

1. Rapid transport to a surgical facility is necessary.
2. The cause of the arrest must be found and specifically treated.
3. Three rescuers are needed to treat the arrest: one to stabilize the neck and ventilate, one to do compressions, and one to find and treat the cause of the arrest.

General Plan of Action

Secure the patient's airway and control the cervical spine. Open the airway with the modified jaw thrust; if there are no respirations, give four quick breaths. If the airway is obstructed, repeat the jaw thrust and try ventilation again. If the airway is still obstructed, attempt to remove the obstruction with your fingers or a laryngoscope and suction; you will need assistance to maintain cervical stabilization. If this is unsuccessful, do abdominal thrusts (the victim must be on a firm surface). If you are still unsuccessful, you may go to cricothyroidotomy or transtracheal jet insufflation (if you are trained and protocols allow). If you are not able to do this surgical procedure, you may do back blows and the Heimlich maneuver. There is a chance of injuring the spine if

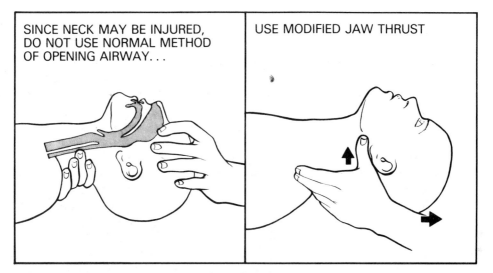

Figure 12-3. Modified jaw thrust.

there is an associated vertebral injury, but this is of less concern if the patient is dying of an airway obstruction. (Desperate situations require desperate measures.)

If the airway is not obstructed, give four quick breaths and then check for the carotid pulse. This can be done without releasing the spine. If no pulse is palpable, you must begin cardiopulmonary resuscitation and prepare for immediate transport. Allow two of your teammates to do the cardiopulmonary resuscitation while you get the monitor and apply the quick-look paddles. If ventricular fibrillation is

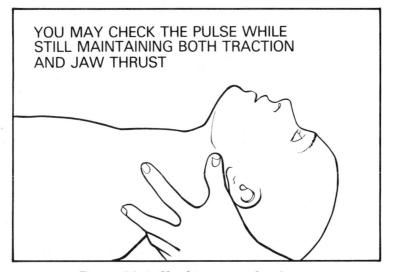

Figure 12-4. Checking carotid pulse.

present, go ahead and defibrillate at 200 watts/sec. Repeat once if not successful. Follow standard ACLS guidelines.

If asystole or EMD is present or if the ventricular fibrillation does not quickly convert to a rhythm with a palpable pulse, you must quickly evaluate and treat the patient for the cause of the arrest. This should be done in the ambulance during transport if possible. You have already treated hypoxia by ventilating with 100% oxygen. You have covered for electric shock and myocardial contusion by standard ACLS protocols. The three conditions you must now rule out are hemorrhagic shock, tension pneumothorax, and pericardial tamponade.

Look at the neck. Are the neck veins flat or distended? Is the trachea midline? Listen to the chest. Are breath sounds present on both sides? If breath sounds are decreased or absent on one side, percuss to see if the side is hyperresonant or dull. Look for obvious bleeding. Look at the abdomen for obvious intra-abdominal bleeding. Look at the pelvis and legs. Are there pelvic or multiple leg fractures?

If there are distended neck veins, decreased breath sounds on one side of the chest, the trachea deviated away from the side of the injury, and hyperresonance to percussion of the chest on the affected side, you can assume that tension pneumothorax is present. Call Medical Control immediately for permission to decompress.

If the neck veins are distended but the trachea is midline and breath sounds are bilateral, you must suspect pericardial tamponade. Apply MAST and attempt to start two large bore intravenous lines. Make all possible haste to the emergency room.

If the neck veins are flat and there is evidence of hemorrhage (decreased breath sounds on one side with dullness on percussion, obvious bleeding, distended abdomen, multiple fractures, or unstable pelvis), you must assume the arrest is secondary to hemorrhagic shock. Apply MAST and attempt to start two large bore intravenous lines. Transport the patient immediately to the emergency room.

Important Points to Remember

1. Cardiac arrest following trauma is usually *not* due to cardiac disease.
2. Do not rely on ACLS protocols alone.
3. Transport the patient rapidly; most procedures must be performed in the ambulance during transport. Do not waste valuable time.
4. Look for and treat the cause of the arrest.
5. You need adequate manpower to handle this situation well: one person to drive the ambulance, one person to stabilize the neck and ventilate, one person to do chest compressions, and one person to diagnose and treat the cause of the arrest.
6. Cardiac arrest in the pregnant victim is treated the same as for other victims. Defibrillation settings and drug dosages are exactly the same.

Chapter 13

"Load-and-Go" Situations

There are certain situations that require hospital treatment within minutes if the victim is to have any chance for survival. When these situations are recognized, the victim should be loaded immediately onto a backboard, transferred to the ambulance, and transported rapidly with lights and siren. Lifesaving procedures may be needed but should be done during transport. Nonlifesaving procedures (such as splinting and bandaging) *must not* hold up transport.

The following are load-and-go situations:

1. Airway obstruction that cannot be quickly relieved by mechanical methods such as suction or forceps
2. Trauma cardiorespiratory arrest
3. Tension pneumothorax
4. Pericardial tamponade
5. Penetrating wounds of the chest with shock
6. Massive hemothorax with shock
7. Head injury with unilaterally dilated pupil
8. Head injury with rapidly deteriorating condition

In all of these cases you must call ahead to have the emergency room and possibly the operating room prepared for your arrival. If a specific surgeon is needed (chest surgeon for numbers 3–6 and neurosurgeon for numbers 7 and 8), have him called before you arrive. Rapid transport is not lifesaving if the necessary surgeon is not available to treat the victim when he arrives.

Chapter 14

Intravenous Cannulation

Resuscitation of the trauma victim very frequently requires the use of drugs. For a drug to be effective in resuscitation, it must not only be available when you need it, but there must be a route available to get it to the part of the body that needs it. The drugs needed most commonly in the trauma victim are oxygen and intravascular fluid. The techniques of providing an airway to get oxygen to the lungs have been covered; now we must consider ways to provide a route to give intravascular fluids. MAST provides a way of shifting part of the available intravascular fluid (blood) from the legs and abdomen to the central circulation, but this fluid still must be replaced before the MAST can be deflated.

Most people tend to **underestimate** the amount of fluid needed to resuscitate the victim in hypovolemic shock. Remember that, generally, symptoms do not appear until 2 to 3 units of blood are lost and you must infuse 3 cc of Ringer's lactate for every 1 cc of blood lost. This means that once symptoms of hemorrhagic shock are present, you are already 3,000 to 4,500 cc of fluid behind. The point should be made here that vasoconstrictors such as metaraminol (Aramine®), norepinephrine (Levophed), or dopamine (Intropin) have no place in the resuscitation of hemorrhagic shock.

Since the purpose of an intravenous line in the trauma victim is almost always volume replacement, you should use IV equipment that will help you accomplish this. The size and length of the IV catheter is very important. Fluid flows fastest through a large diameter *short* tube. Thus, you should use IV tubing without the extension set (it can be added later) and use a short over the needle cannula of 14- or 16-gauge. In the same length of time, twice as much fluid will flow through a 14-gauge cannula as through a 16-gauge (and three times as much as through an 18-gauge). You should also always use the plastic IV containers rather than the glass. Not only are they less likely to break, but you can wrap a blood pressure cuff around them, pump them up to 300 mm Hg, and increase the flow rate to three to four times the normal. All of these things can be very important in someone who is already in deep shock when you arrive.

If the patient is in shock or is actively bleeding, you must start an intravenous line **quickly**. The route you choose is very important. Sub-

153

clavian vein cannulation is technically difficult, has potential for serious complications, and often takes repeated attempts to be successful. It should be left to the more controlled environment of the emergency room. A large peripheral vein is the site of choice in the field. You must develop the skill to quickly find and cannulate two different sites. The patient who is already hypotensive should have MAST applied before you attempt intravenous cannulation. MAST is quicker to apply, replaces blood rather than just fluid, and usually makes it easier to find and cannulate a peripheral vein.

Choice of Site for Intravenous Cannulation

The first choice is the large veins of the lower arm or antecubital space. If you cannot find a suitable vein in these areas, you should use the external jugular vein or the femoral vein.

I. **External Jugular Vein**
This is a useful, though usually forgotten, route for volume replacement.

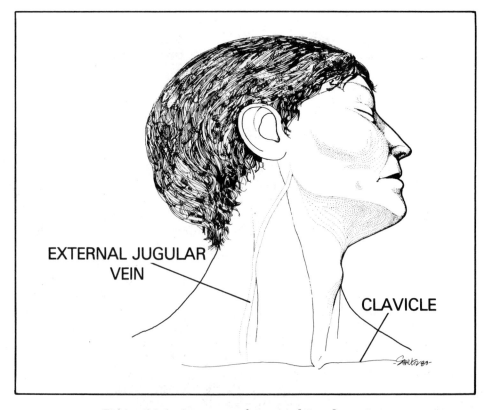

Figure 14-1. Anatomy of external jugular vein.

A. Surface anatomy: The external jugular vein runs in a line from the angle of the jaw to the junction of the medial and middle thirds of the clavicle. It is usually easily visible through the skin and can be made prominent by pressing on it just above the clavicle. It runs into the subclavian vein.

B. Technique of cannulation
   1. The victim must be in the supine position and preferably head down to distend the vein and prevent air embolism.
   2. If there is no danger of cervical spine injury, you should turn the patient's head to the opposite side. If there is a danger of cervical spine injury, the head must not be turned, but rather must be stabilized by one rescuer while the IV is started.
   3. Quickly prepare the skin with antiseptic and then align the cannula with the vein. The needle will be pointing at the clavicle at about the junction of the middle and medial thirds.
   4. With one finger press on the vein just above the clavicle. This should make the vein more prominent.
   5. Insert the needle into the vein at about the midportion and cannulate in the usual way.
   6. If not done already, draw a 30-cc sample of blood and store it in red and purple stopper tubes.
   7. Tape the line down securely. If there is danger of a cervical spine injury, a cervical collar can be applied over the IV site.

II. **Femoral Vein**
The veins of the leg have generally not been used as IV sites because of the danger of developing thrombophlebitis and subsequent pulmonary emboli. This fear is not justified if the vein is used only temporarily for resuscitation. If the femoral vein is used, the IV should be changed in the emergency room to a more suitable location.

A. The **advantages** of the femoral vein are as follows.
   1. It is a large vein that goes directly into the inferior cava.
   2. Usually, it is easy to cannulate.

B. The **disadvantages** are as follows.
   1. It cannot be done with MAST in place.
   2. It cannot be seen through the skin, so the pulsation of the femoral artery must be used to locate it. This can be difficult if the patient is hypotensive.
   3. If the victim has abdominal trauma, the inferior vena cava may be injured. Replacement fluids may simply leak out into the abdomen.

C. Anatomy: The femoral vein is in the femoral sheath that runs through the femoral triangle of the upper leg. In the middle

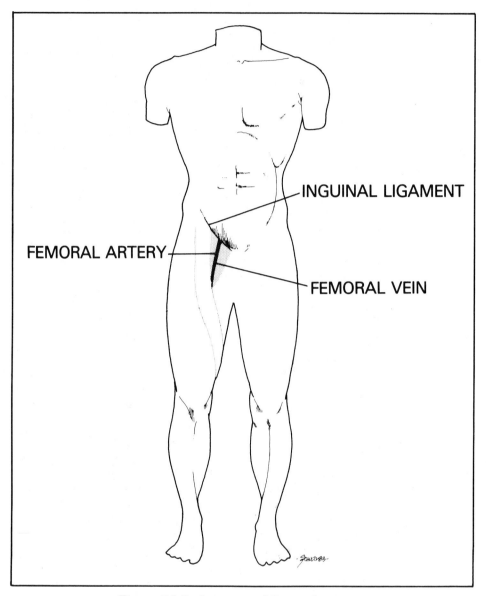

Figure 14-2. Anatomy of femoral vein.

of the femoral triangle it lies medial to the femoral nerve
and artery.

D. Technique of cannulation

1. The patient should be supine but should not be head
    down.

2. Identify your landmarks. Find the superior iliac spine and
    the symphysis pubica. Find the midpoint of a line be-
    tween those two points and then feel for the femoral
    pulse two finger breadths below that point.

3. Prepare this area with antiseptic.
4. Holding the fingers of one hand on the femoral artery, insert the cannula with syringe attached just medial and in a cephalad direction. It should be inserted parallel to the long axis of the body.
5. Insert the cannula at a 45-degree angle to the skin, as-pirating as you go. You may have to go the full length of the needle, then withdraw slowly while gently aspirating.
6. When blood appears, complete your cannulation in the usual way and tape securely to the skin. Withdraw 30 cc of blood before attaching IV tubing.
7. If you inadvertently puncture the femoral artery, you will see bright red blood fill the syringe under some pres-sure. There is no harm done. Simply withdraw the needle (you may get your 30 cc of blood first) and reinsert the cannula just medial to this site. You should hold pressure on the arterial puncture site for 5 minutes.
8. Remember, if you start a femoral IV line, it must be changed to another site in the emergency room when the patient is stabilized.

Upper Airway Management I

Objectives

The objectives of this skill station are as follows:

1. To learn various manual methods of opening the airway
2. To learn how to suction the airway
3. To learn how to insert a nasopharyngeal and oropharyngeal airway
4. To learn how to use the pocket mask
5. To learn how to use the bag-valve mask

Procedures

I. **Manual Techniques to Open the Airway**
   A. Modified jaw thrust
      1. Place your hands on either side of the neck at the base of the skull.

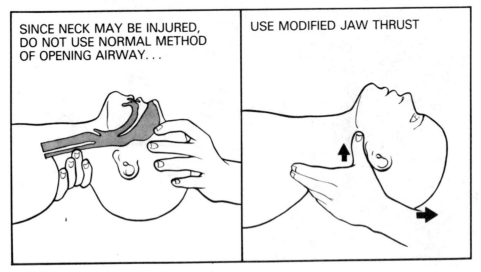

SINCE NECK MAY BE INJURED, DO NOT USE NORMAL METHOD OF OPENING AIRWAY...

USE MODIFIED JAW THRUST

Figure S1-1. Modified jaw thrust.

159

      2. While maintaining in-line traction on the neck, push up on the angles of the mandible with your thumbs.

  B. Jaw thrust (two-man procedure)
      1. Have your partner stabilize the neck in a neutral position.
      2. Using the index and middle fingers of each hand, grasp the angles of the jaw just below the ears.
      3. Gently lift.

  C. Chin lift (two-man procedure)
      1. Have your partner stabilize the neck in a neutral position.
      2. Place the fingers of one hand under the anterior mandible.
      3. Grasp the chin below the lower lip with the thumb.
      4. Lift gently.

II. **Suctioning the Airway**
  A. Attach the suction tubing to the device.
  B. Turn the device on and test the portable suction machine.
  C. Insert the suction tube through the nose, pharynx, or ET tube without activating the suction.
  D. Activate the suction and withdraw the tube.
  E. Repeat the procedure as necessary.
  F. Use the technique of turning a patient with possible cervical spine trauma to clear secretions or vomitus from the upper airway.

III. **Insertion of Pharyngeal Airways**
  A. Nasopharyngeal airway
      1. Choose the appropriate size.

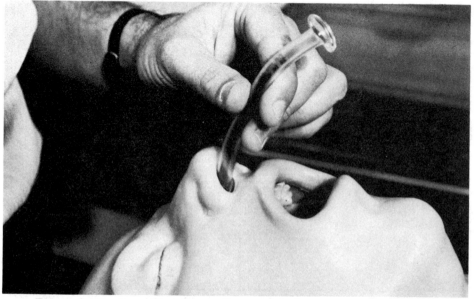

Figure S1-2a. Insertion of nasopharyngeal airway into right nostril.

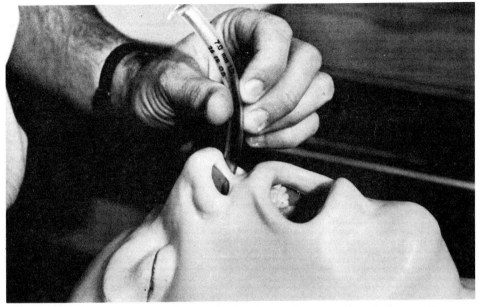

Figure S1-2b. Insertion of nasopharyngeal airway into left nostril.

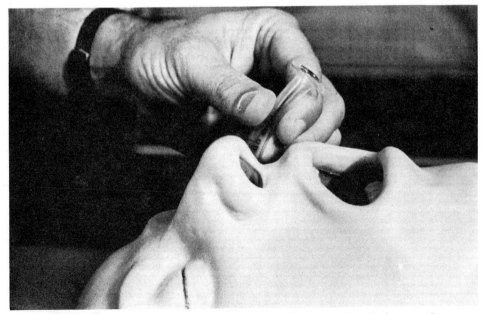

Figure S1-2c. Insertion of nasopharyngeal airway into left nostril.

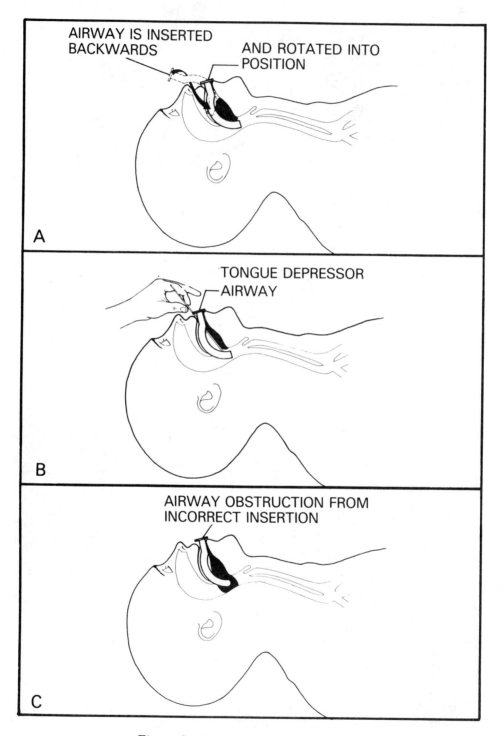

Figure S1-3. Insertion of oral airway.

2. Lubricate the tube.
3. Insert it straight back through the nose with the beveled edge of the airway toward the septum.

B. Oropharyngeal airway
   1. Choose the appropriate size.
   2. Open the airway.
      a. Scissor maneuver
      b. Jaw lift
      c. Tongue blade
   3. Insert the airway gently without pushing the tongue back into the pharynx.
      a. Insert the airway upside down and rotate it into place.
      b. Insert the airway under direct vision using the tongue blade.

IV. **Use of Pocket Mask with Supplemental Oxygen**
   A. Have your partner stabilize the neck in a neutral position (or apply a good stabilization device).
   B. Connect the oxygen tubing to the oxygen cylinder and the mask.
   C. Open the oxygen cylinder and set the flow rate at 12 L/min.
   D. Open the airway.
   E. Insert the oral airway properly.
   F. Place the mask on the face and establish a good seal.

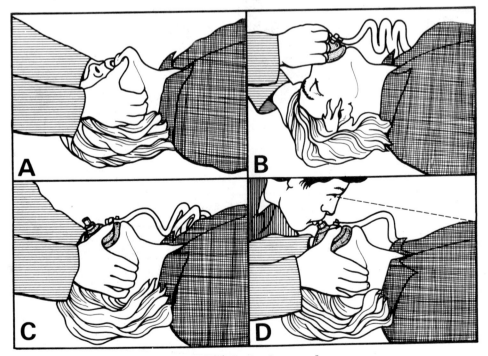

Figure S1-4. Pocket mask.

G. Ventilate mouth to mask with a sufficient volume (about 800 cc) to cause the green light to come on in the recording mannequin.

V. **Use of Bag-Valve Mask**

A. Stabilize the neck with a suitable device.
B. Connect the oxygen tubing to the bag-valve system and oxygen cylinder.
C. Attach the oxygen reservoir to the bag-valve mask.
D. Open the oxygen cylinder and set the flow rate at 12 L/min.
E. Select the proper size mask and attach it to the bag-valve device.
F. Open the airway.
G. Insert the oral airway properly.
H. Place the mask on the face and have your partner establish and maintain a good seal.
I. Ventilate with a sufficient volume (about 800 cc) to cause the green light to come on in the recording mannequin. Use both hands.

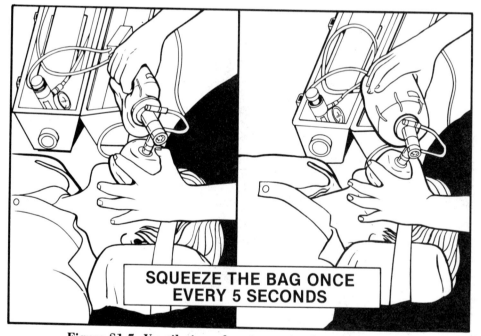

Figure S1-5. Ventilation of patient using bag-valve mask.

Airway Management II

Objectives

The objectives of this skill station are as follows:

1. To learn adult endotracheal intubation
2. To learn to insert the esophageal gastric tube airway (EGTA)
3. To learn to intubate the trachea while the EGTA is in place
4. To learn infant endotracheal intubation

Procedures

I. **Adult Endotracheal Intubation**
   A. Stabilize the neck in a neutral position from below (done by your partner).
   B. Assume that ventilation is in progress.
   C. Be sure that a suction apparatus is available and functioning.
   D. Select the correct size ET tube. Insert a wire guide, attach a 10-cc syringe, and test the cuff.
   E. Connect the laryngoscope blade and handle. Test the light.
   F. Hold the laryngoscope in your left hand.
   G. Insert the laryngoscope blade in the right side of the mouth, moving the tongue to the left.
   H. Visualize the vocal cords.
   I. Insert the ET tube.
   J. Check the placement of the ET tube by ventilating through the tube while listening for bilateral breath sounds with a stethoscope. Observe the patient to see if the chest rises with ventilation.
   K. Inflate the cuff with 4 to 6 cc of air.
   L. Secure the tube.

II. **Insertion of EGTA**
   A. Stabilize the neck in a neutral position from below (done by your partner).
   B. Assume that ventilation is in progress.

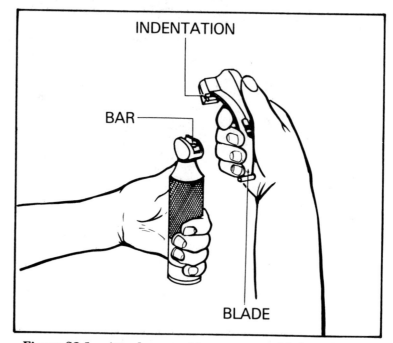

Figure S2-1a. Attachment of laryngoscope blade to handle.

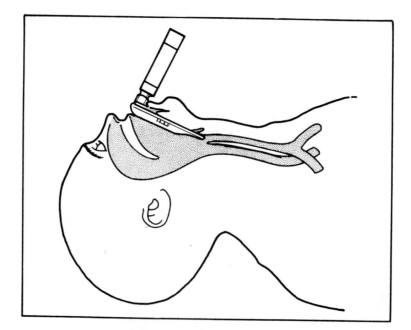

Figure S2-1b. Laryngoscope: straight blade.

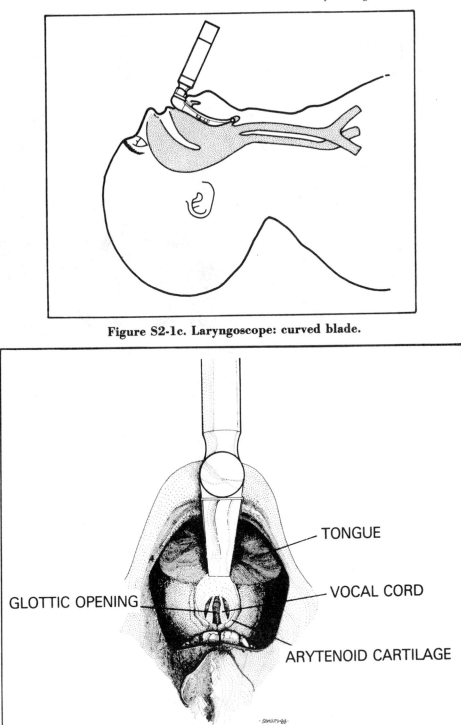

Figure S2-1c. Laryngoscope: curved blade.

TONGUE

VOCAL CORD

GLOTTIC OPENING

ARYTENOID CARTILAGE

Figure S2-1d. Insertion of straight blade.

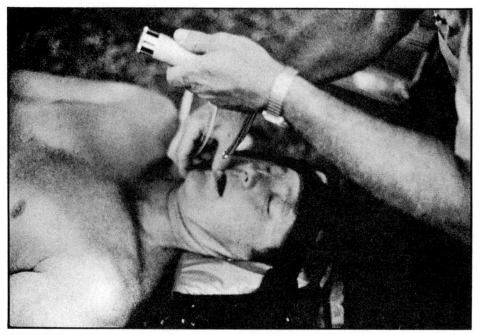

Figure S2-1e. Insertion of straight blade.

C. Suction the pharynx.

D. Attach the mask to the EGTA.

E. Attach a 30-cc syringe to the EGTA and test the balloon.

F. Grasp the jaw between the thumb and index finger and lift upward—do not hyperextend the neck.

G. Insert the tube into the mouth with the curve of the tube matching the curve of the pharynx.

H. Advance the tube into the esophagus until the mask seals firmly on the face.

I. Ventilate while listening for breath sounds with a stethoscope: observe to see that the chest rises.

J. Inflate the cuff with 30 cc of air.

K. Check for breath sounds again.

III. **Tracheal Intubation with EGTA in Place**

A. Start with the EGTA in place and the neck stabilized in a neutral position from below.

B. Suction the pharynx.

C. Intubate the trachea using the correct procedure.

D. Test for adequate ventilation.

E. Remove the EGTA.

F. Apply a cervical stabilization device.

IV. **Infant Intubation**

A. Have your partner stabilize the neck in a neutral position.

B. Assume that ventilation is in progress.

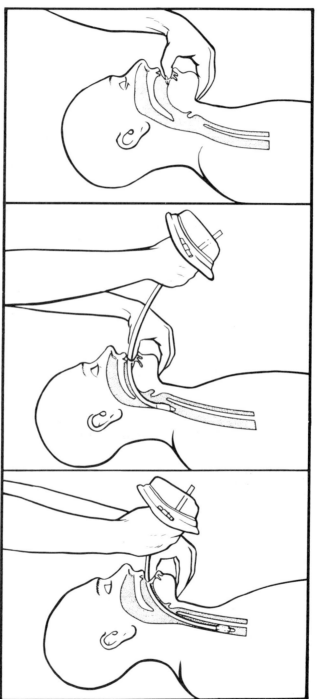

Figure S2-2a. Insertion of esophageal airway.

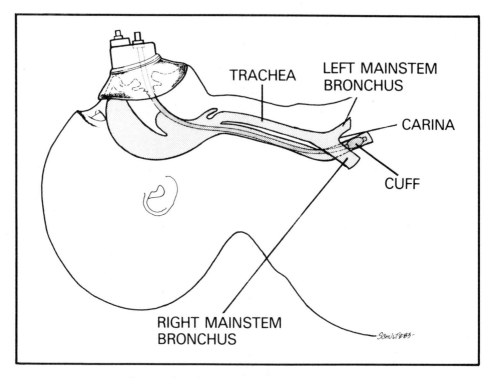

TRACHEA

LEFT MAINSTEM BRONCHUS

CARINA

CUFF

RIGHT MAINSTEM BRONCHUS

Figure S2-2b. Final position of EGTA.

C.   Be sure suction apparatus is available and functioning.
D.   Select the correct size ET tube and insert the wire guide.
E.   Connect the laryngoscope blade and handle. Test the light.
F.   Hold the laryngoscope in your left hand.
G.   Insert the laryngoscope blade in the right side of the mouth, moving the tongue to the left.
H.   Visualize the vocal cords.
 I.   Insert the ET tube.
J.   Check for placement of the tube by listening for bilateral breath sounds while ventilating.
K.   Secure the tube.

Management of Tension Pneumothorax

Objectives

The objectives of this skill station are as follows:

1. To learn the indications for emergency decompression of a tension pneumothorax
2. To learn the technique of needle decompression of a tension pneumothorax
3. To learn the complications of needle decompression of a tension pneumothorax

The following outline covers these points.

I. **Indication for Needle Decompression of Tension Pneumothorax**
   This is to be done only when specifically ordered by your Medical Control physician. It is only for a patient with a tension pneumothorax and whose condition is rapidly deteriorating in spite of oxygen and ventilatory assistance.

II. **Procedure for Needle Decompression of Tension Pneumothorax**
   A. Assess the patient to be sure his condition is due to a tension pneumothorax.
      1. Poor ventilation
      2. Neck vein distention
      3. Tracheal deviation away from the side of the injury
      4. Absent or decreased breath sounds on the affected side
      5. Hyperresonance to percussion on the affected side
      6. Shock
   B. Give the patient high flow oxygen.
   C. Identify the fifth intercostal space in the midaxillary line (the nipple is usually over the fifth rib) on the same side as the pneumothorax.
   D. Quickly prepare the area with a Betadine® swab.
   E. Make a flutter-valve by inserting a #14 gauge over the needle

171

catheter through the cut off finger of a rubber glove (or a condom).

F. Insert the catheter into the skin over the fifth rib and direct it just over the top of the rib (superior border) into the interspace.

G. Insert the catheter through the parietal pleura until air exits through the flutter-valve. It should exit under pressure.

H. Remove the needle and leave the plastic cannula in place until it is replaced by a chest tube at the hospital.

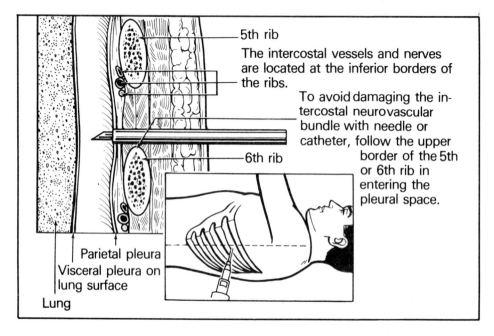

5th rib

The intercostal vessels and nerves are located at the inferior borders of the ribs.

To avoid damaging the intercostal neurovascular bundle with needle or catheter, follow the upper border of the 5th or 6th rib in entering the pleural space.

6th rib

Parietal pleura
Visceral pleura on lung surface
Lung

Figure S3-1. Needle decompression of tension pneumothorax.

III. **Complications of Needle Aspiration of Tension Pneumothorax**

A. Laceration of intercostal vessel with resultant hemorrhage: The intercostal artery and vein run around the inferior margin of each rib. Poor placement of the aspirating needle can lacerate one of these vessels.

B. Creation of a pneumothorax if not already present: If your assessment was not correct, you may give the patient a pneumothorax when you insert the needle into the chest.

C. Laceration of the lung: Poor technique or inappropriate insertion (no pneumothorax present) can cause laceration of the lung, causing bleeding and more air leak.

D. Infection: This can occur if the skin was not prepped.

Application of Military Anti-Shock Trousers (MAST)

Objectives

The objectives of this skill station are as follows:

1. To learn and practice the proper method of applying and inflating MAST
2. To learn and practice the proper method of deflating and re-moving MAST
3. To learn (and to be able to discuss) the indications and contrain-dications for the use of MAST

Caution: If these trousers are applied to live models, do *not* inflate them; they may cause elevations in the blood pressure.

Procedure

I. **Application**
   A. Evaluate the patient (including his vital signs). Leave the blood pressure cuff on his arm.
   B. Unfold the trousers and lay them flat on a long spine board or the stretcher.
   C. Maintaining immobility of the spine, place the patient on the stretcher so that the top of the garment is just below the lowest rib.
   D. Wrap the trousers around the left leg and fasten the Velcro® strips.
   E. Wrap the trousers around the right leg and fasten the Velcro strips.
   F. Wrap the abdominal compartment around the abdomen and fasten the Velcro strips. Be sure the top of the garment is below the bottom ribs.

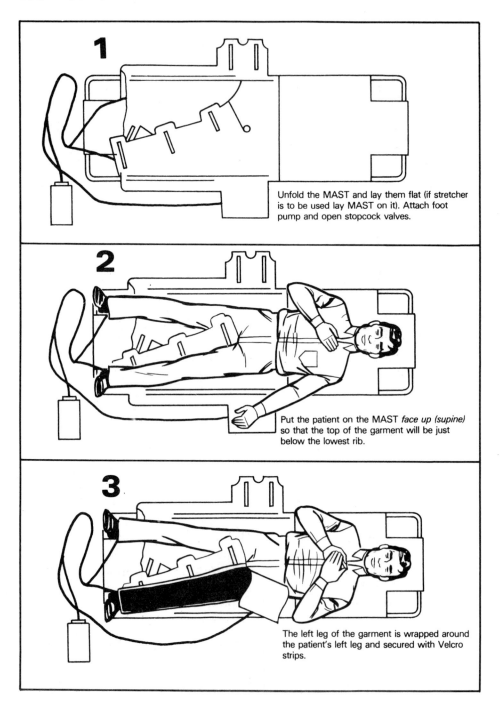

1 Unfold the MAST and lay them flat (if stretcher is to be used lay MAST on it). Attach foot pump and open stopcock valves.

2 Put the patient on the MAST *face up (supine)* so that the top of the garment will be just below the lowest rib.

3 The left leg of the garment is wrapped around the patient's left leg and secured with Velcro strips.

Figure S4-1. Application of the MAST.

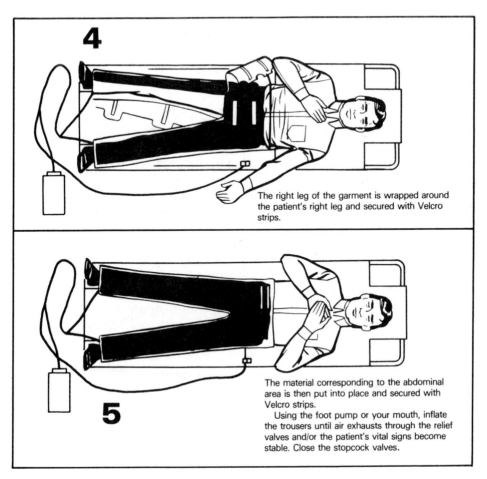

4

The right leg of the garment is wrapped around the patient's right leg and secured with Velcro strips.

5

The material corresponding to the abdominal area is then put into place and secured with Velcro strips.

Using the foot pump or your mouth, inflate the trousers until air exhausts through the relief valves and/or the patient's vital signs become stable. Close the stopcock valves.

Figure S4-1 (cont.). Application of the MAST.

G. If you are going to use the foot pump, attach the air tubes to the connections on the trousers. It is quicker to blow up the compartments with your mouth; if you prefer to do it this way, you do not need the foot pump, air tubes, or gauges at all.

II. **Inflation of Trousers**

A. Recheck and record the vital signs.

B. Inflate the leg compartments while monitoring the blood pressure. If the blood pressure is not in the 100 to 110 mm Hg range, inflate the abdominal compartment.

C. When the patient's blood pressure is adequate (100 to 110 mg Hg), turn the stopcocks to hold the pressure.

D. Remember, it is not the pressure in the trousers you are monitoring but the pressure in the patient.

E. Continue monitoring the patient's blood pressure, adding pressure to the trousers as needed.

III. **Deflation of Trousers**

Note: Before deflation occurs, you must insert two large bore IVs and give sufficient volume of fluids and/or blood to replace the volume lost from hemorrhage.

A. Record the patient's vital signs.

B. Obtain permission to deflate the trousers **from a physician knowledgeable in their use.**

C. Slowly deflate the abdominal compartment while monitoring the patient's blood pressure.

D. If the blood pressure drops 5 mm Hg or more, you must stop deflation and infuse more fluid or blood until the vital signs stabilize again (this usually requires at least 200 cc).

E. Proceed from the abdominal compartment to the right leg and then left leg with your deflation, continuously monitoring the blood pressure and stopping to infuse fluid when a drop of 5 mm Hg occurs.

F. If the patient experiences a sudden precipitous drop in blood pressure while you are deflating, stop and reinflate the garment.

IV. **Application of MAST to a Victim Requiring a Traction Splint**

A. Have your partner hold traction on the fractured leg.

B. Unfold the trousers and lay them flat on a long spine board.

C. Log roll the victim, holding traction on the injured leg and keeping the neck stabilized.

D. Slide the spine board and trousers under the victim so that the top of the trousers is just below the lowest rib. If the victim is already on a spine board, you may simply unfold the trousers and slide them under the victim while maintaining traction on the injured leg.

E. Wrap the trousers around the injured leg and fasten the Velcro strips.

F. Wrap the trousers around the other leg and fasten the Velcro strips.

G. Wrap the abdominal compartment around the abdomen and fasten the Velcro strips. Be sure the top of the garment is below the bottom ribs.

H. Apply a traction splint (Thomas, Hare, Sager, or Klippel) *over* the trousers. Attach the straps and apply traction.

I. Inflate the trousers in the usual sequence.

Critical Points

1. Remove the trousers only in the hospital setting unless pulmonary edema is precipitated by application.
2. Inflate the trousers until a systolic blood pressure of 100 to 110 mm Hg is obtained.
3. Monitor vital signs frequently.
4. Always start two IVs and replacement fluids.
5. During deflation, a blood pressure drop of 5 mm Hg signals that deflation must stop until more fluids are given.
6. *Never* allow deflation of the MAST by personnel inexperienced in its use.
7. Never deflate the MAST without an adequate volume replacement immediately available and a good intravenous route already established.
8. Never deflate the entire garment at once.
9. Never deflate the legs before the abdomen.
10. Do not let personnel holding scissors near the garment.
11. If necessary, patients may go to surgery with the garment in place.

Review

I. **Indications for Use of MAST**
   A. Systolic blood pressure less than 80 mm Hg
   B. Systolic blood pressure of 100 or less associated with other symptoms of shock
   C. Neurogenic shock
   D. Pelvic fractures
   E. Fractures of lower extremities
   F. Spinal shock
   G. Massive abdominal bleeding

II. **Contraindications for Use of MAST**
   A. Absolute: pulmonary edema
   B. Conditional
      1. Pregnancy: may use leg compartments
      2. Abdominal injury with protruding viscera: use leg compartments

Helmet Removal and Head Trauma Assessment

Objectives

The objectives of this skill station are as follows:

1. To learn to remove a helmet without injuring the spine
2. To learn the proper way to evaluate for head trauma

Procedures

I. **Procedure to Remove a Helmet from a Patient with a Possible Cervical Spine Injury**
   A. The first rescuer positions himself above or behind the victim, places his hands on each side of the helmet, and applies traction in-line with the spine. He should grasp the patient at the angles of his mandible at the same time so that the traction is applied to the victim's head through his hands rather than through the chin strap.
   B. The second rescuer positions himself to the side of the victim and removes or cuts the chin strap.
   C. The second rescuer then assumes the in-line traction on the spine by placing one hand under the neck at the occiput and the other hand on the anterior neck with the thumb pressing on one angle of the mandible and the index and middle fingers pressing on the other angle of the mandible. The first rescuer releases his traction and holds the helmet only.
   D. The first rescuer now removes the helmet by pulling out laterally on each side to clear the ears and then up to remove. Full face helmets will have to be tilted back to clear the nose (tilt the helmet, not the head). If the victim has glasses on, the first rescuer should remove them through the visual opening before removing the full face helmet. The second rescuer maintains steady traction during this procedure.

179

E. After removal of the helmet, the first rescuer takes over the traction again by grasping the head on either side with his fingers holding the angle of the jaw and the occiput.

F. The second rescuer now applies a suitable cervical immobilization device.

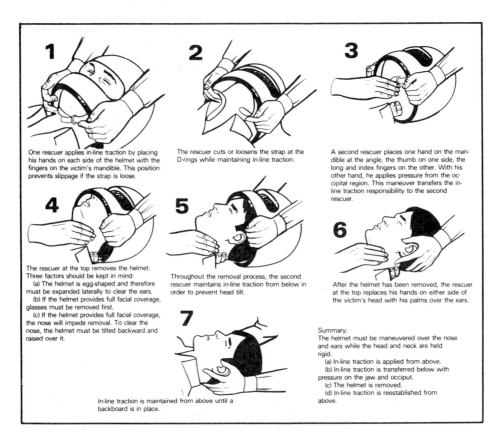

1 One rescuer applies in-line traction by placing his hands on each side of the helmet with the fingers on the victim's mandible. This position prevents slippage if the strap is loose.

2 The rescuer cuts or loosens the strap at the D-rings while maintaining in-line traction.

3 A second rescuer places one hand on the mandible at the angle, the thumb on one side, the long and index fingers on the other. With his other hand, he applies pressure from the occipital region. This maneuver transfers the in-line traction responsibility to the second rescuer.

4 The rescuer at the top removes the helmet. Three factors should be kept in mind:
(a) The helmet is egg-shaped and therefore must be expanded laterally to clear the ears.
(b) If the helmet provides full facial coverage, glasses must be removed first.
(c) If the helmet provides full facial coverage, the nose will impede removal. To clear the nose, the helmet must be tilted backward and raised over it.

5 Throughout the removal process, the second rescuer maintains in-line traction from below in order to prevent head tilt.

6 After the helmet has been removed, the rescuer at the top replaces his hands on either side of the victim's head with his palms over the ears.

7 In-line traction is maintained from above until a backboard is in place.

Summary:
The helmet must be maneuvered over the nose and ears while the head and neck are held rigid.
(a) In-line traction is applied from above.
(b) In-line traction is transferred below with pressure on the jaw and occiput.
(c) The helmet is removed.
(d) In-line traction is reestablished from above.

Figure S5-1. Helmet removal from injured patient.

II. **Alternate Procedure for Removal of Helmet**
This has the advantage that one rescuer maintains traction during the whole procedure.

A. The first rescuer positions himself above or behind the victim and places his hands on each side of the neck at the base of the skull. He applies steady in-line traction with the neck in a neutral position. He may use his thumbs to perform a modified jaw thrust while doing this.

B. The second rescuer positions himself over or to the side of the victim and removes or cuts the chin strap.

C. The second rescuer now removes the helmet by pulling out laterally on each side to clear the ears and then up to remove.

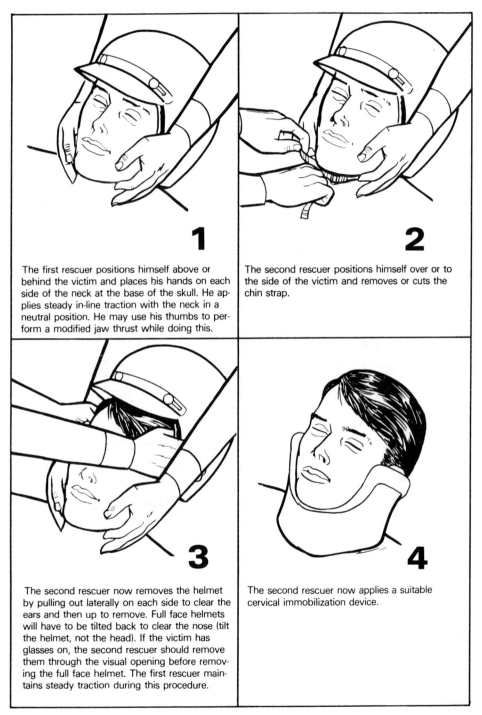

1

The first rescuer positions himself above or behind the victim and places his hands on each side of the neck at the base of the skull. He applies steady in-line traction with the neck in a neutral position. He may use his thumbs to perform a modified jaw thrust while doing this.

2

The second rescuer positions himself over or to the side of the victim and removes or cuts the chin strap.

3

The second rescuer now removes the helmet by pulling out laterally on each side to clear the ears and then up to remove. Full face helmets will have to be tilted back to clear the nose (tilt the helmet, not the head). If the victim has glasses on, the second rescuer should remove them through the visual opening before removing the full face helmet. The first rescuer maintains steady traction during this procedure.

4

The second rescuer now applies a suitable cervical immobilization device.

Figure S5-2. Alternate method for removal of helmet.

Full face helmets will have to be tilted back to clear the nose (tilt the helmet, not the head). If the victim has glasses on, the second rescuer should remove them through the visual opening before removing the full face helmet. The first rescuer maintains steady traction during this procedure.

D. The second rescuer now applies a suitable cervical immobilization device.

III. **Procedure for Rapid Assessment of Head Trauma**

A. Assess the airway and apply traction to the cervical spine.

B. Assess breathing and circulation.

C. Stop any bleeding.

D. Obtain vital signs and assess for shock: note the level of consciousness.

E. Splint fractures (you may apply a cervical collar) and palpate the cervical spine at this time.

F. Secondary survey

1. Carefully palpate the scalp for lacerations. If lacerations are present, palpate to determine if there is a depressed skull fracture associated with them.

2. Take note of bleeding from the nose or ears.

3. Take note of the signs of basilar skull fracture (raccoon eyes, Battle's sign).

4. Palpate the bones of the face for possible fracture.

5. Examine pupil size and reaction to light.

6. Apply dressings to lacerations.

7. Quickly assess motor function and sensation in arms and legs.

8. Complete secondary survey.

G. Notify Medical Control.

H. Continuously monitor: Recheck the level of consciousness, vital signs, pupil size, and reaction every 5 minutes.

I. Transport the patient on a backboard with cervical spine immobilization.

Spinal Immobilization

Objectives

The objectives of this skill station are as follows:

1. To learn when to use spinal immobilization
2. To learn the correct technique of spinal immobilization with a short backboard
3. To learn the correct technique of spinal immobilization with a long backboard

The following outline covers the above objectives.

I. **Who Should Have Spinal Immobilization?**
    A. Any victim of trauma with obvious neurological deficit such as paralysis, weakness, or paresthesia (numbness or tingling)
    B. Any victim of trauma who complains of pain in the head, neck, or back
    C. Any victim of trauma who is unconscious
    D. Any victim of trauma who may have injury to the spine but in whom evaluation is difficult due to altered mental status (e.g., drugs, alcohol)
    E. Any unconscious patient who may have been subjected to trauma
    F. Any trauma victim with facial or head injuries
    G. When in doubt, immobilize.

II. **When to Immobilize**
Patients requiring immobilization must have it done before they are moved at all. In the case of an automobile accident, the victim must be immobilized before he is removed from the wreckage. More movement is involved in extrication than at any other time, so immobilization of neck and spine must be accomplished before beginning extrication.

III. **Technique of Spinal Immobilization Using the Short Backboard**
This device is for use in the patient who is in a position (such as an automobile) that does not allow use of the long backboard. There are several different devices of this type; some devices have

different strapping mechanisms from the one explained here. You must become familiar with the equipment you will employ before using it in the field.

A. Remember that the routine priorities of evaluation and management of the trauma victim are done before the immobilization devices go on.

B. One rescuer must, if possible, station himself behind the victim, place his hands on either side of the victim's head, and apply gentle traction. The neck is held in a neutral position. This step is part of the ABCs of evaluation. It is done at the same time that you begin evaluation of the airway.

C. When you have the patient stable enough to begin splinting, you must apply a cervical collar (Philadelphia or comparable semirigid device). If you have enough manpower, this can be done while someone else is doing the ABCs of evaluation and management.

D. Position the backboard behind the victim. The first rescuer continues to hold traction while the short backboard is being maneuvered into place. The victim may have to be moved forward to get the backboard in place; great care must be taken that moves are coordinated so as to support the neck and back.

E. Secure the victim to the board: There are usually two straps for this. Bring each strap over a leg, down between both legs, back around the outside of the same leg, and then across the chest, then attach them to the opposite upper straps that were brought across the shoulders.

F. Tighten the straps until the victim is held securely.

G. Secure the victim's head to the board by cravats around the forehead. The first rescuer may now release traction. A Kerlix roll is placed under the neck for support.

H. Transfer the victim to a long spine board: Turn the patient so his back is to the opening through which he is to be removed. Someone must support his legs so that the upper legs remain at a 90-degree angle to the torso. Position the long spine board through the opening until it is behind the victim. Lower the victim back onto the long spine board and slide the victim and short spine board up into position on the long spine board. Loosen the straps on the short board and allow the patient's legs to extend out flat and then retighten the straps. Now secure him to the long board with straps, and secure his head with sandbags or a Bashaw device. When he is secured in this way, it is possible to turn the whole board up on its side if he has to vomit. He will remain securely immobilized.

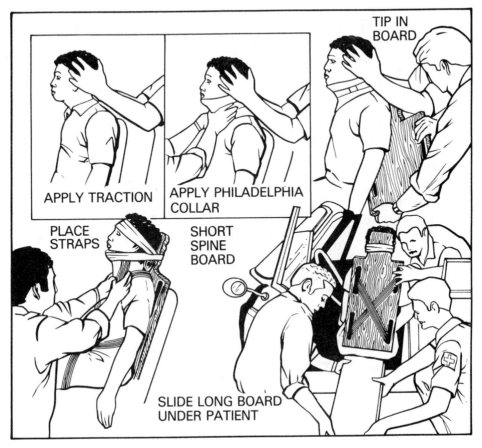

Figure S6-1. Use of the short backboard.

I.   Points to remember
   1.   When you are placing the straps around the legs on a male, do not catch the genitals in the straps.
   2.   Do not use the short board as a "handle" to move the patient. Move both patient and board as a unit.
   3.   When you are attaching the horizontal straps (long spine board) around a woman, place the upper strap above her breasts, not across them.
   4.   When you are applying the lower horizontal strap on a pregnant woman, see that it is low enough so as not to injure the fetus.
   5.   Injuries may force you to modify how you attach the straps.
   6.   The patient must be secured well enough to have no motion of the spine if the board is turned on its side.

IV. **Technique for Using the Long Spine Board**
This is used without the short board when the patient is supine or can be safely transferred to a supine position without the use of the short board.

A. Perform routine priority assessment and management.

B. Hold traction on the head and spine (in a neutral position) while a cervical collar is applied. Continue holding traction while the patient is transferred to the long board.

C. Log roll the patient to either side and position the long board behind him.

D. Pad the board at the neck, lumbar area, and knees.

E. Roll the patient back onto the board and secure him with straps.

F. Secure the head with sandbags and cravats or with a device such as the Bashaw device.

Extremity Immobilization

Objectives

The objectives for this skill station are as follows:

1. To learn to use splints
    a. traction splints (Thomas, Hare, Klippel)
    b. soft splints
    c. air splints
    d. rigid splints
2. To learn to immobilize fractures or dislocations
    a. fractured femur
    b. fractured or dislocated hip
    c. fractured or dislocated knee or elbow
    d. fractured tibia / fibula
    e. fractured humerus
    f. fractured clavicle
    g. dislocated shoulder
    h. fractured wrist or forearm
    i. fractured ankle or foot

Procedures

I. **Traction Splints**
    These splints are used most often for fractured femurs. They require two rescuers for application. The victim should already be on a stretcher or backboard.
    A. Thomas splint (half-ring splint)
        1. The first rescuer supports the leg while the second rescuer cuts away the clothing and removes the shoe and sock to assess distal circulation and sensation.
        2. Position the splint under the injured leg. The ring goes down and the short side goes to the inside of the leg. Slide the ring snugly up against the ischial tuberosity.

3. Position two support straps above the knee and two below the knee.
4. Attach the top ring strap.
5. Apply padding to the foot and ankle.
6. Apply the traction hitch around the ankle and foot.
7. Apply gentle traction by hand.
8. Attach the traction hitch to the end of the splint.
9. Increase traction by Spanish windlass action using a stick or tongue depressors.
10. Release manual traction and reassess circulation and sensation.
11. Support the end of the splint so that there is no pressure on the heel.

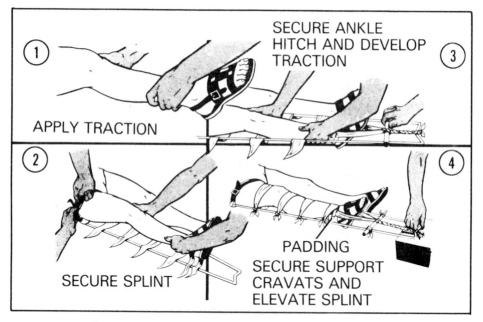

Figure S7-1a. Applying a traction (Thomas) splint.

B. Hare splint
1. The first rescuer supports the leg while the second rescuer cuts away the clothing and removes the shoe and sock to assess sensation and circulation.
2. Position the splint under the injured leg. The ring goes down and the short side goes to the inside of the leg. Slide the ring snugly up against the ischial tuberosity.
3. Position two support straps above the knee and two below the knee.
4. Attach the heel rest.
5. Attach the top strap.

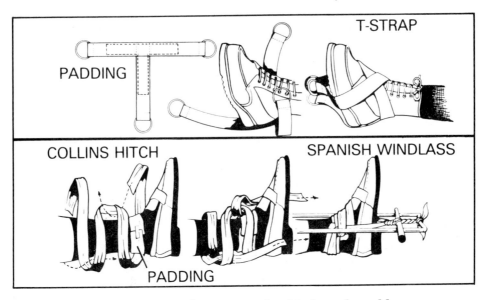

T-STRAP

PADDING

COLLINS HITCH

SPANISH WINDLASS

PADDING

Figure S7-1b. Applying a traction hitch to the ankle.

6. Apply the padded traction hitch to the ankle and foot.
7. Apply gentle manual traction.
8. Attach the traction hitch to the windlass by way of the S-hook.
9. Turn the ratchet until the correct tension is applied and then release manual traction.
10. Reassess circulation and sensation.
11. Attach support straps around the leg with Velcro straps.
12. To release traction, pull the ratchet knob outward and then slowly turn to loosen.

C. Klippel splint
1. The first rescuer supports the leg while the second rescuer cuts away the clothing and removes the shoe and sock to assess distal circulation and sensation.
2. Using the good leg as a guide, pull the splint out to the current length.
3. Turn the footplate up by pushing to the side and then turning it.
4. Turn the heel rest down by pushing in both knobs simultaneously and then turning.
5. Maintain gentle traction and support. Slide the splint under the leg (ring turned down) until the ring is snugly against the ischial tuberosity.
6. Position two support straps above the knee and two below the knee.
7. Attach the top ring strap.

8. Push the footplate up against the sole of the foot. Push the two release levers to shorten the splint.
9. Apply padding to the foot and ankle.
10. Bring the traction hitch up under the ankle and then cross the two straps over the foot, around the footplate, and back over the foot where they attach by Velcro fasteners.
11. Exert manual traction and then extend the splint by pulling on the two rails until correct tension is obtained.
12. Release manual traction.
13. Reassess circulation and sensation.
14. Attach the support straps around the leg with Velcro fasteners.

II. **Immobilization**
   A. Fractured hip
      1. Evaluation reveals pain and tenderness over the hip.
      2. Evaluate the distal pulses and sensation.
      3. Place the patient on a spine board.
      4. Place a blanket between the legs for padding.
      5. Bind the legs together by way of straps. The straps for securing the patient to the spine board may be enough, but you may have to use an ACE™ wrap for more support.
   B. Dislocated hip: Most hip dislocations are posterior. The leg

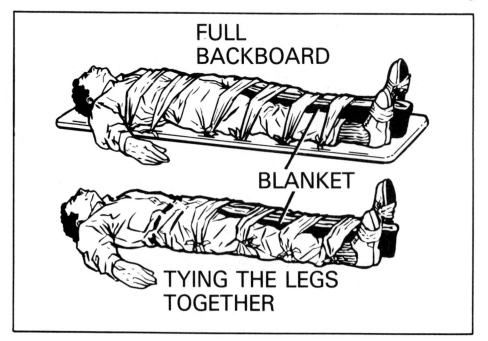

FULL BACKBOARD

BLANKET

TYING THE LEGS TOGETHER

Figure S7-2. Hip fracture.

will be flexed at the hip and knee and rotated inward. There is extreme pain.

1. Evaluate the distal pulses and sensation.
2. Place the patient on a backboard with a pillow or rolled blanket supporting the leg in the most comfortable position.
3. Transport the patient quickly.

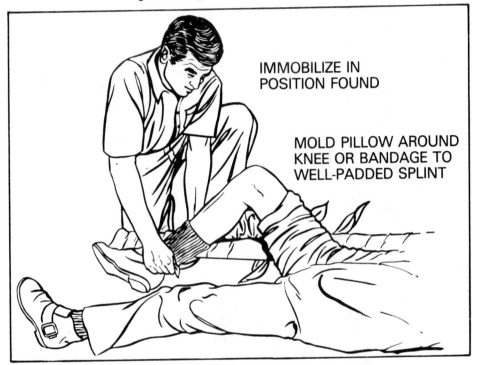

IMMOBILIZE IN POSITION FOUND

MOLD PILLOW AROUND KNEE OR BANDAGE TO WELL-PADDED SPLINT

Figure S7-3. Splinting posterior dislocation of the hip.

C. Fractured or dislocated knee: This may be straight or flexed. Injury to nerves and arteries is common.
1. Evaluate for circulation and sensation.
2. Splint in the position you find the leg. If the leg is straight, use a long leg air splint, MAST, or a traction splint (use only gentle traction).
3. If the leg is flexed, support it with a pillow or rolled blanket. The patient may be more comfortable on his side with the injured knee supported on a pillow. A rigid splint may be used to stabilize the leg more.
D. Fractured or dislocated elbow: This injury also may occur with the arm straight or flexed. Vascular or neurological injury is frequent. Splinting of the arm should be in the position in which you find it.

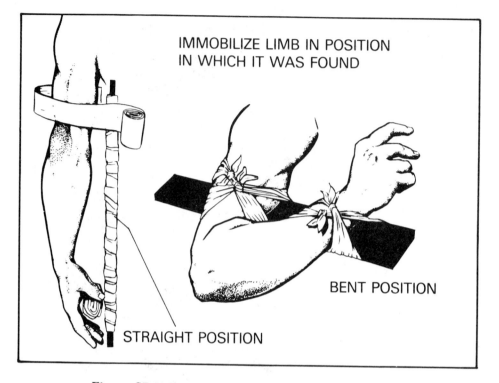

IMMOBILIZE LIMB IN POSITION
IN WHICH IT WAS FOUND

BENT POSITION

STRAIGHT POSITION

Figure S7-4. Fractures or dislocations of the elbow.

1. Evaluate for circulation and sensation.
2. If the arm is flexed, support it with a sling and swathe, bend a metal ladder splint to fit (pad well), or attach a padded board splint across the upper and lower arm to stabilize it.
3. If the arm is straight, use a padded board or ladder splint. Secure it with a sling or ACE wrap from the axilla to the wrist.
4. Check the circulation when the splint is applied.

E. Fractured tibia / fibula
   1. Proximal fracture:
      a. Evaluate for circulation and sensation.
      b. Splint the leg with a traction splint (see section on traction splints).
   2. Distal fracture:
      a. Evaluate for circulation and sensation.
      b. Splint the leg with a short leg air splint or padded board splint. You may use a traction splint.

F. Fractured ankle or foot
   1. Evaluate circulation and sensation.

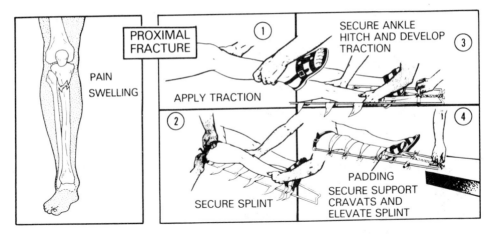

Figure S7-5a. Splinting lower leg fractures.
Proximal fracture—traction splint.

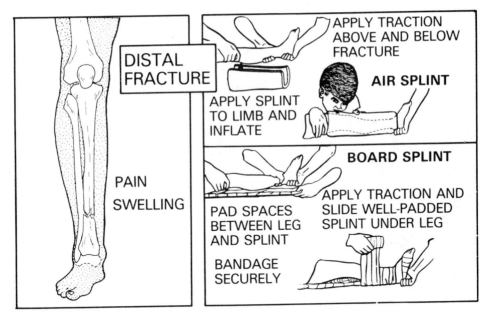

Figure S7-5b. Splinting lower leg fractures.
Distal fracture—air splint or board splint.

  2. Splint the fracture with a short leg air splint or pillow
      splint.
G. Fractured clavicle
  1. Evaluate sensation and circulation.
  2. Immobilize the clavicle with a sling and swathe.
H. Dislocated shoulder: This may also be a fracture of the head
    of the humerus.
  1. Evaluate distal sensation and circulation.

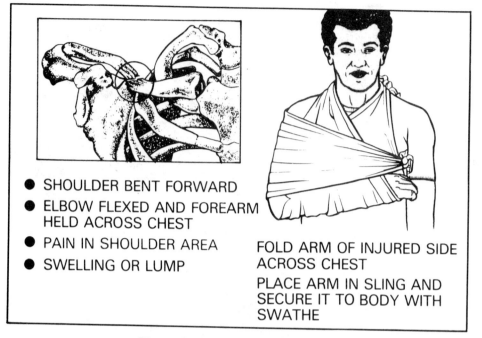

- SHOULDER BENT FORWARD
- ELBOW FLEXED AND FOREARM HELD ACROSS CHEST
- PAIN IN SHOULDER AREA
- SWELLING OR LUMP

FOLD ARM OF INJURED SIDE ACROSS CHEST

PLACE ARM IN SLING AND SECURE IT TO BODY WITH SWATHE

Figure S7-6. Fractured clavicle.

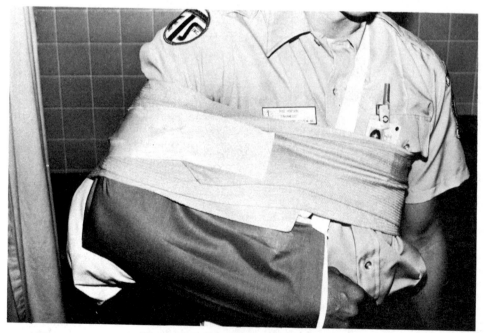

Figure S7-7. Dislocated shoulder.

    2. Immobilize the shoulder in the most comfortable position using a towel, blanket, or pillow along with a sling and swathe.

I. Fractured upper arm
    1. Evaluate sensation and circulation.
    2. Support the arm with a sling and swathe.

J. Fractured forearm or wrist
    1. Evaluate sensation and circulation.
    2. Immobilize the fracture with a cylinder air splint, cardboard splint, padded board, or ladder splint and then support the arm / wrist with a sling. Put a roll of kling in the palm to hold the hand in the position of function.

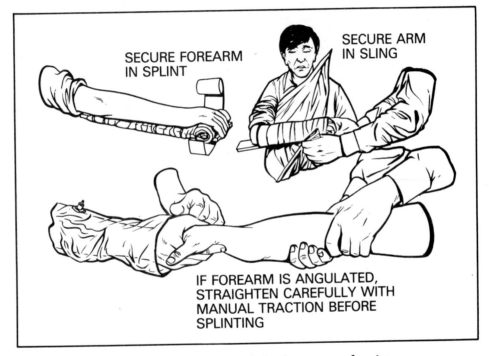

SECURE FOREARM IN SPLINT

SECURE ARM IN SLING

IF FOREARM IS ANGULATED, STRAIGHTEN CAREFULLY WITH MANUAL TRACTION BEFORE SPLINTING

Figure S7-8. Fractures of the forearm and wrist.

Intravenous Cannulation

It is expected that all students of this course are familiar by now with the technique of inserting an intravenous cannula in the veins of the lower arm or antecubital space, so only other sites will be discussed here.

Objectives

The objectives of this skill station are as follows:

1. To learn the technique of cannulation of the external jugular vein
2. To learn the technique of cannulation of the femoral vein

Procedures

I. **Cannulation of External Jugular Vein**
   A. The victim must be in the supine position, preferably head down, to distend the vein and prevent air embolism.
   B. If there is no danger of cervical spine injury, you should turn the patient's head to the opposite side. If there is a danger of cervical spine injury, the head must not be turned but rather must be stabilized by one rescuer while the IV is started.
   C. Quickly prepare the skin with an antiseptic and then align the cannula with the vein. The needle will be pointing at the clavicle at about the junction of the middle and medial thirds.
   D. With one finger press on the vein just above the clavicle. This should make the vein more prominent.
   E. Insert the needle into the vein at about the midportion and cannulate in the usual way.
   F. If it was not done already, draw a 30 cc sample of blood and store it in red and purple stopped tubes.
   G. Tape down the line securely. If there is a danger of a cervical spine injury, a cervical collar can be applied over the IV site.

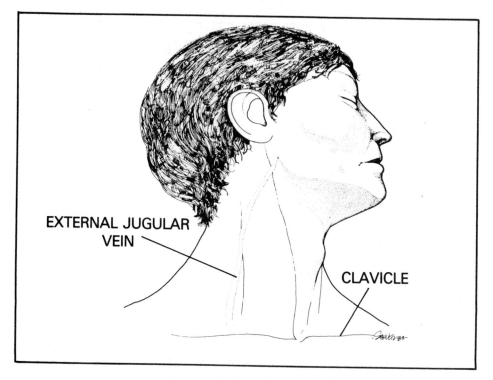

EXTERNAL JUGULAR VEIN

CLAVICLE

Figure S8-1. Anatomy of external jugular vein.

II. Cannulation of Femoral Vein

A. The patient should be supine but should not be head down.

B. Identify your landmarks. Find the superior iliac spine and the symphysis pubica. Find the midpoint of a line between those two points and then feel for the femoral pulse two finger breadths below that point.

C. Prepare this area with an antiseptic.

D. Holding the fingers of one hand on the femoral artery, insert the cannula with syringe attached just medial and in a cephalad direction. It should be inserted parallel to the long axis of the body.

E. Insert the cannula at a 45-degree angle to the skin, aspirating as you go. You may have to go to the full length of the needle and then withdraw slowly while aspirating gently.

F. When blood appears, complete your cannulation in the usual way and tape it securely to the skin. Withdraw 30 cc of blood before attaching the IV tubing.

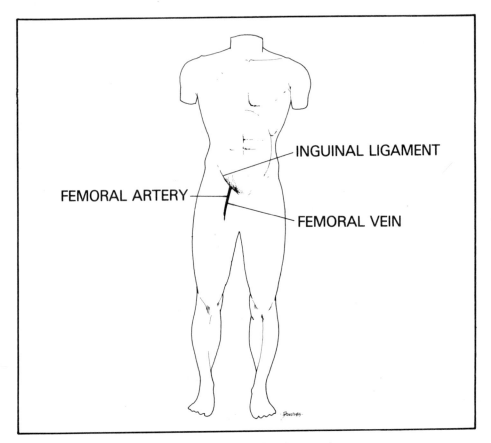

Figure S8-2. Anatomy of femoral vein.

Patient Evaluation and Management

Objective

The objective of this skill station is to practice the proper sequence of evaluation and management of the multiple trauma victim.

Procedure

The instructor will demonstrate how to properly evaluate and manage a multiple trauma victim using the techniques and principles described in the Basic Trauma Life Support course.

A short written scenario will be used along with a model (to act as the victim). The students will be allowed to practice the management of simulated trauma situations using appropriate rescue and stabilization equipment.

Index